I0782038

WHO KILLED NIA JOHNES ?

Elisabeth Link, M.D

WHO KILLED NIA JOHNES ?

*

A Medical Mystery

Elisabeth Link, M.D

First published in the United States of America
by Monasteria Press LLC, San Francisco
© Monasteria Press 2023

Every effort has been made in providing up-to-date information about infectious diseases and other medical conditions in this book, which is in accord with accepted standards and medical practices at the time of publication. Nevertheless, the author and publisher can make no warranty that the information contained herein is totally free from error, not least because accepted standards and practices are constantly changing. The author and publisher therefore disclaim any and all liability for direct or consequential damages resulting from the use of information contained in this book.

Paperback ISBN: 978-1-958277-04-1
Hardback ISBN: 978-1-958277-00-3
eBook ISBN: 978-1-958277-03-4

Cover design by Paul Palmer-Edwards

DEDICATION

For my students

Acclaim for Elizabeth Link

"A medical mystery novel with interesting characters and captivating story arc. I was hooked from page one."

"An excellent read from a talented writer. Highly recommend!"

"A medical detective story that makes you smarter. I wished I had this in medical school."

"Elizabeth Link reveals the truth about academic medicine. Too many of us met Dr. Robinson in real life."

"Inspiring female protagonist. Great plot, great role models."

"My new favorite writer."

"In the end you'll see who's fake, who's true,
and who would risk it all just for you."

—Unknown

CONTENTS

WHO KILLED NIA JOHNES?

*

A Medical Mystery

Elisabeth Link, M.D.

Who killed Nia Johnes ?

PROLOGUE

Silicon Valley University of Evolutionary Computation (SUEC) was established in 2025 in a secluded location in the hills above Redwood City, California. SUEC realized a new model of collaboration between major tech companies and the state of California to develop cutting-edge technologies within the framework of a research-intensive university. Evolutionary computation (EC) uses principles from biological development to solve computational problems. Reversed EC uses computer algorithms to advance biological development. An initial set of solutions is generated and iteratively updated by small random changes until a target performance has been achieved.

Many of the innovations developed and explored at SUEC are years ahead of what is available anywhere else. Therefore, SUEC has attracted the most famous faculty and the brightest students from around the world. To provide convenient medical services, SUEC owns a hospital in nearby Redwood City that is open to the public and provides medical emergency care, general medical care, and a variety of medical specialty services for both adult and pediatric patients.

As the center of technological innovation in the world, generating billions of dollars in donations and revenue, SUEC is a constant target for spies, thieves, and other criminals. Therefore, the university has a large security team and sophisticated surveillance and protection systems to protect its workers and work products. In addition, the US government has deployed undercover FBI and CIA agents to protect SUEC's assets of national interest and identify any activities that might impair the national security.

In 2032, FBI special agents Angus Weber and Terrel Wright, undercover CIA agent Dr. Annya Segond, and SUEC radiologist Dr. Lili Pham worked together to find stolen brain-computer interfaces and save the University from a bomb threat. Since then, life at the University has been calm and idyllic. SUEC researchers and clinician-scientists are focusing on their work and creating their next groundbreaking discoveries amidst the beautiful scenery of the sunny California redwood hills.

Who killed Nia Johnes ?

- 1 -

NIA

The Threat
Tuesday, May 24, 2033, 10:55 p.m.

Nia was brushing her teeth when the cell phone rang. She checked the time. 10:55 p.m. *Who would call so late?* She put more pressure on the toothbrush to clean her front teeth. She liked the minty taste.

The phone rang again.

Nia looked into the mirror. Her eyes looked tired. She would ignore this stupid phone. She could not speak right now anyways.

The phone kept ringing.

She spat the toothpaste foam into the sink, then gargled.

The phone kept ringing.

Nia got so irritated that she swallowed some of the foam. She cursed and glanced at the display: Annya Segond. *The emergency physician from the hospital?* Dr. Segond had treated her for a pneumonia some time ago. But Nia had no clinical problem right now. Why did Dr. Segond call her? Were any of her friends injured? Or did she know about the infections?

Nia grabbed the phone.

It stopped ringing.

Now, that was annoying!

Nia turned off the lights in the bathroom and walked into the bedroom, where her cozy queen bed waited for her. The day had been hectic. She looked forward to crawling under the neatly folded flowered bedsheet and plunging her head into the silky-soft pillows. She stepped into her walk-in closet, looking for her pajamas.

The phone started ringing again.

Nia cursed again. But this time, she picked up right away.

"Hello?"

"Hello, this is Dr. Annya Segond, the emergency physician at

SUEC hospital. Is this Nia Johnes?"

"Yes, this is she."

"I am glad to hear your voice! Are you okay?"

"Of course, I am. Why are you asking?"

"Nia, I have a request that might sound a little strange to you. Every apartment at SUEC has a security system. I need you to activate it right now, turn off all lights, and close all the curtains—do it now, please."

Strange indeed. Nia looked around. Her small apartment looked peaceful and sleepy, just like her. "The security system is already activated. I always turn it on when I come home at night. What is going on?"

"Good. Now turn off the lights and close all the curtains."

Nia shook her head. She looked at the window. It was dark outside. Dim light from streetlamps illuminated a small path and a volleyball court behind the building. There was nobody. In the distance was a sea of redwood trees moving gently with the evening breeze, like a fairytale. Nia pushed a button beside the window. The roller blinds emerged from each side with a purring sound.

"Nia, are you still there?" Dr. Segond asked.

"I closed the bedroom curtains. The living room does not have any. What is this all about?"

"Nia, the SUEC security team informed me that you are in danger. I worked with the security team for many years, and since I live in the building next to yours, they asked me to check on you. In fact, they thought that you were already injured."

"I'm fine. Perhaps you called the wrong person?"

"You are Dr. Nia Johnes—Johnes with an "h"? A PhD in infectious diseases and postdoctoral fellow in Dr. Walker-Díaz's lab?"

"Yes, this is me."

"Is it possible that someone wants to hurt you, Nia?"

Nia hesitated for just a second. "I don't think so."

"Well, the SUEC security team thinks so. They intercepted a communication that suggested that you *were* already compromised."

"Who said that? And I told you, I'm fine. Perhaps this is just some sick, racist prank!"

"I am afraid this is a real threat, Nia. At least, we have to take it very seriously."

Nia started to feel uneasy. "You scare me!"

"Please stay calm. I will come by to check on you now. Stay where you are, and do not touch anything. Do not eat or drink anything. Do not open the door. I will be at your apartment in a few minutes."

"Thank you, Dr. Segond. Hopefully, this can all be resolved."

"Please don't let your guard down, Nia. I will be there shortly."

Nia hung up the phone. Her mind was spinning. Dr. Segond had treated her several times for minor illnesses at SUEC hospital. Nia remembered the ER physician as a pretty middle-aged woman who was professional, competent, and trustworthy. But she also remembered some rumors last year that Dr. Segond had been pursued by the FBI. Who knew? Perhaps Dr. Segond was the threat here. But when she had met Dr. Segond in the hospital, Nia had found her to be a very likable, experienced physician. Nia had recovered from her pneumonia in no time.

Perhaps someone else had just *pretended* to be Dr. Segond? Any woman could have called and pretended to be her. Nia tried to suppress her nagging fear. Could someone know about her discovery? Whoever the woman was, perhaps she just wanted to come to her apartment in the middle of the night and destroy the files.

Nia stepped into the living room, where her laptop sat on a large desk besides the window. She grabbed it and stuffed it into her backpack. She walked towards the entryway of the apartment and slipped into her sneakers. *Just in case.*

There was a faint ruffling noise. Nia looked around, trying to locate it. Did it come from the door? She stared at the plain, paneled front door. There was the sound again. *Has Dr. Segond arrived already? No, she could not arrive that fast. And if it were her, she would surely ring the doorbell or say something.*

Nia stood perfectly still as she watched the apartment door, about two meters in front of her. *Did the door handle move down?* She squinted her eyes. *The door handle is moving!*

Nia held her breath as she stared at the door. Her heart pounded up to her eardrums as the door opened slowly. She tiptoed backwards, away from the entrance.

The door opened some more until the deadbolt clicked in. Four fingers in a dark leather glove appeared in the small gap between the door and the doorframe, then moved upwards towards the metal bolt, carefully palpating the culprit that was blocking the door.

Nia jumped around. She grabbed the backpack, opened the living room window, and hopped through the window frame onto the decorative balcony in front of it. The balcony planks squeaked under her weight, and the balcony tilted downwards. It was on the second floor.

Nia looked down. Below her was the outdoor volleyball court. Nia had played many games there with the SUEC sports team. The floor had built-in shock absorbers, so it should be possible to jump. Perhaps. Nia adjusted the backpack on her back, then carefully climbed over the railing of the balcony, which continued to sink under her weight.

A loud blowing sound filled the air. Nia looked back and saw the door fling wide open. The alarm system kicked in, and a loud siren ended the silence of the night.

A person in a dark motorcycle suit and helmet stood in the doorframe, scanning the room, then looking at Nia behind the open window. They quickly raised their left arm and pointed a gun at her.

Nia heard a high-pitched noise beside her right ear. She cowered down, grabbing the railing, then letting her body slide down and leaping off the building. She landed on the soft floor of the volleyball court, jumped up, and ran as fast as her feet would take her.

- 2 -

ANNYA

Tuberculosis
Tuesday, May 24, 2033, 11:05 p.m.

Dr. Annya Segond walked with long strides to the apartment building. She heard a loud siren and started to run. One by one, the dark square windows in the apartment building lit up. Annya noticed heads appearing in some of them, checking the perimeter of their honeycombs for the source of the nuisance.

The entrance door of the building was wide open. Annya raced through it and up the stairs, taking two stairs at once. There were several students in the hallway, some in their street clothes, others in pajamas. Several had pulled out their phones and filmed the scene. Then the siren stopped.

Annya arrived at a demolished apartment door. A security guard rushed past her and blocked the entrance. Annya stopped and showed him her SUEC faculty ID. "I am part of the security team at SUEC. I live on campus and received a call from the security manager to check on Dr. Nia Johnes."

The guard looked her up and down. "Our team will be here momentarily."

Annya sighed. With her ponytail and jogging outfit, she probably looked like the students in the hallway. "I *am* part of the security team!" She flashed her CIA ID.

The guard slowly pulled his phone out of his pocket and talked with someone in a low voice while staring at Annya. Then, he hung up the phone and stepped aside. "I am afraid you are too late. Mrs. Johnes left through her window a few minutes ago. Witnesses heard gunshots here." The guard waved towards the apartment.

Annya pointed at the name tag at the door. "It is Dr. Johnes," she said calmly.

"I'm not sure it matters if it's Mrs. Dead or Dr. Dead." The guard said with a chuckle. "You can wait inside. Please do not touch anything."

Annya looked at him with a stern gaze. The guard rolled his eyes. *I hope he finds a brain back there,* she thought as she passed him and stepped into the apartment.

Annya felt as if she were walking into a tropical island garden. The room was packed with potted palm trees, ferns, philodendrons, and orchids. To her right was a huge potted bamboo palm, a rattan wicker couch with cream cushions, and a fluted side table on a turquoise rug. Above the couch was a large framed ocean beach poster. To the left of the couch were large windows with a decorative balcony in front of them. One of the windows was wide open, sending a cool breeze into the room. The railing of the balcony appeared unusually tilted.

Annya stepped to the window and looked at the volleyball court below it. Two security guards walked across the field, checking all directions with flashlights.

Annya turned back to the apartment. To her left was a raw wood desk with a pile of printed documents. The desk was flanked on each side by large Yucca palm trees. The guard at the door looked at her again. "Don't touch anything!"

Annya made a mental note to check out the files on the desk later. In the distance, hallway doors shut. Apparently, the spectators had decided to return to their rooms. *Good.*

Annya turned around and checked out the bedroom and bathroom. As expected, they were empty. She heard voices at the door and turned. A handsome black man in a perfectly ironed gray suit walked into the apartment and greeted her. "Annya. Long time no see."

"Hello, Terrel," Annya responded. "How comes the FBI is interested in a runaway researcher?"

"Well, we have some intel that this case might threaten national security. If an SUEC employee who researches infectious diseases is pursued by a criminal, we want to make sure that all bacteria and viruses stay in the lab and don't get lost."

"That is very thoughtful of you!" Annya smiled wryly. "How about chasing the criminal?"

"Three policemen are pursuing the scientist and a man with a gun right now. They will let me know when they've found them. Meanwhile, I wanted to see what was so interesting here."

"Perhaps the scientist herself?"

"There is always something that a criminal wants. And we might as well find it here."

Annya nodded.

"How did you get involved?" Terrel asked. "I thought you retired from the CIA after the events last year."

"You know I cannot comment on that. I am fully committed to my work as an emergency physician now. But can I *really* retire from the CIA?"

Terrel looked at her with a tilted head. "Probably not."

"I received a call from the SUEC security team tonight. They had overheard a conversation on a walkway in the SUEC village. There are fiber-optic cables buried underneath the ground that are listening to pedestrians who walk past."

"Wow, that sounds like a Big Brother story."

"Yea, initial versions of this technology, called the big glass microphone, have been tested at Stanford and the V&A in London. SUEC has substantially advanced this technology such that it can recognize human voices and screen for specific words that might indicate crimes."

"Interesting! And it detected a concerning conversation about Nia Johnes today?"

"Yes, indeed. At 11:30 p.m. tonight, a man asked if Nia Johnes had been eliminated. A woman responded that Nia was incapacitated and would be dead before midnight. This conversation initiated an alert, and our security team called me to check on her because I live right next door. Unfortunately, she had left when I arrived." Annya pointed at the open window.

"Our team is tracking her cell phone," Terrel explained. "We will find her very soon. Do you know her? Why would anyone want to kill her?"

"I saw her at the hospital several times, but I do not know her otherwise, and I have no idea what this is about."

Terrel looked around. "Let's see if we can find any clues here."

"I would suggest starting with that desk." Annya pointed at the piles of files.

Terrel nodded. He stepped towards the desk and flipped through the files. Annya looked over his shoulder. There were multiple research publications, several medical bills, a registration receipt for a scientific conference, a birthday card, two folders with numbers on them, a gift certificate for a local restaurant, and an invitation for a dibling party.

"Dibling? Is that a typo?" Terrel took photos of the documents.

"Diblings are donor-conceived siblings," Annya explained. "People who were conceived from a sperm or egg donation can find half-siblings who were conceived from the same donor through online registries and DNA testing kits. Dibling parties are organized to introduce these half-siblings to each other."

"Fascinating!" Terrel made a note in his notebook, then opened one of the folders on the desk. It contained paper prints of medical imaging studies. "Do you know if this is a CT scan or an MRI?" he asked Annya, holding up the first printout.

"This is a CT scan—computed tomography," Annya responded. "The bones are very dense. This is because the x-rays cannot penetrate the bone very well. On an MRI, they would be dark."

"Does this CT scan show any abnormalities?"

"Yes, this scan is very abnormal. You can see multiple cavitating lesions in the left upper lung. And there are enlarged lymph nodes around the hilum." Annya pointed to the abnormalities.

"What does that mean?"

"I believe this is pneumonia. I remember that we treated Nia for coccidiomycosis, a fungus infection. Perhaps this is her own CT scan."

Terrel looked at her. "Can you call your radiologist friend Lili Pham to find out more details? She has access to all imaging files at SUEC hospital and can probably look this up quickly."

"Well, it is almost midnight. Do you want to wake Lili up for this? Nia recovered completely from her pneumonia. So, if this is her imaging study, it is not current. Her infection has resolved."

"She could have developed a new infection."

"In principle, but in that case, she would have come to me for another round of treatment. I did not see her recently in the clinic."

"Our team got intel that an unusually high number of infections were recorded at SUEC hospital over the past few months. Now, we are finding medical images of infections on the desk of an SUEC scientist who is being chased by a shooter. Perhaps the images in this folder can help us understand what is going on. Please call your friend."

Annya sighed. Terrel was as inquisitive and relentless as usual.

"And please turn the speakerphone on so that I can hear what she has to say."

Lili answered after the second ring. "Hello?"

"Hi, Lili, this is Annya. I'm sorry to disturb you so late."

"No worries. I'm on call tonight. How can I help? Do you have a consult for me?"

"Well, kind of. I am with FBI Agent Terrel Wright at a crime scene on campus. You might remember him from the FBI investigation at SUEC last year."

"Of course, I remember him."

"We are at an apartment of a young scientist who's disappeared."

"Oh, no! Again?"

"Well, this scientist jumped out of the window, apparently pursued by a man with a gun. Witnesses heard gunshots and saw a man in a dark suit running after her. We searched the apartment and found medical imaging studies on her desk that seem to show infections. Presumably, this is something that she has been working on. Could you have a look and let us know what kind of infection this might be?"

Annya took a snapshot with her phone and sent several of the CT images over to Lili through a secure SUEC online portal.

"Well, it is difficult to make a diagnosis from a few snapshots. What I see here are cavitary lesions of the lung with thick rims and enlarged hilar lymph nodes."

Annya smiled. "That's what I told Terrel. Could it be coccidiomycosis?"

"As you know, radiologists cannot replace mycology or histology analyses. There's always a differential diagnosis. Cavitary lesions in the lungs can be seen in patients with bacterial or fungal infections, among others. But if you suspect this diagnosis clinically, then the imaging findings here would be consistent with a coccidiomycosis."

"Hello, Lili, this is Terrel. You can access the medical images from SUEC hospital from your home, right?"

"Hello, Terrel, long time no hear! Yes, I can."

"Could you please check if the images that we sent to you were images of Nia Johnes?"

"Sure. Is this okay with HIPAA, the Health Insurance Portability and Accountability Act that protects patient privacy?"

"Yes, the FBI can overturn HIPAA in matters of national security and life-and-death scenarios."

"I remember that from our interactions last year. Give me just a minute. Can you spell the name?"

"N-i-a J-o-h-n-e-s."

There was a typing sound in the background. After a while, Lili's voice returned. "You are right. The images are from Nia Johnes. They were obtained a few months ago. There's another follow-up study, which is normal. So, this infection resolved."

Terrel pulled up another file from Nia's desk and handed them to Annya. "I found more images."

Annya took another snapshot and sent them over to Lili.

"Well, this is a CT scan of the chest which shows severe pneumonia," Lili explained. "There are multiple pulmonary nodules in a tree-in-bud distribution."

"Tree-in-bud?" Terrel asked.

"It means that the nodules are found at the end of the vessels, like a budding tree. This infection has spread via the blood vessels. There is also a large pulmonary consolidation in the left lung, a pleural effusion and an abscess around the spine."

Terrel said, "Lili, can you check if these images were from Nia as well?"

"This is definitely a different patient."

"There are more images in this file," Annya said. "I am sending them over. It looks like a CT and MRI of the spine of the same patient."

"Got them! This looks like severe osteomyelitis."

"What's that?" Terrel asked.

"Osteomyelitis is an infection of the bones," Lili explained. "Three subsequent vertebral bodies are involved. The one in the middle is almost completely collapsed. The infection has caused a large abscess in front of the infected vertebral bodies. This is almost certainly tuberculosis."

"I'm glad we called you!" Annya said.

"As mentioned, there are always differential diagnoses. You would want to confirm this diagnosis with microbiological tests."

"Thank you, Lili!"

"Is there anything else that the images tell you?" Terrel asked.

"If this is indeed TB, then this is a young patient—a teenager or young adult. The infection is spread through the blood. Young patients have vessels that supply the intervertebral disks, and I see involvement of the disks here. In older patients, there is sparse blood supply to the disks, and they are typically spared."

"Lili, I assume there are few patients with such severe TB infection at SUEC these days. Could you identify this patient?"

"If you have a search warrant, I could ask our infectious-disease team to provide me with a list of patients with TB in the last two years or so and check if these images belong to any of them."

"I will get you that," Terrel said.

"This was very helpful. Thank you, Lili!" Annya said.

"Any time! Let me know if I can help with anything else."

Annya looked at both folders on Nia's desk. The folder with Nia's images was marked as #1, and the folder of the patient with tuberculosis was marked as #3. "Can you find a number #2 ?" she asked.

Terrel sifted through the pile again. "Nope."

"It's interesting what is not here," Annya said.

Terrel finished the thought. "A computer!"

They both looked around the apartment but could not find a computer anywhere.

"Either Nia or the man with the gun must have taken it!"

The guard at the door came into the room. "They found the girl," he said to Terrel.

- 3 -

NIA

The Secret
Tuesday, May 24, 2033, 11:10 p.m.

Nia raced down the University promenade, towards the parking lot. The path was dimly lit by streetlamps, but she knew the way. She had walked it up and down hundreds of times.

There were footsteps behind her. Whenever her sneakers hit the ground, she heard an echo behind her—shoes hitting the pavement, coming closer. She started to hear heavy breathing sounds behind her. She did not dare to look back. *Run!* she thought. *I must be faster!*

To her right, Nia heard the alarm sirens from the SUEC valley. To her left was thick forest. Should she jump into the woods? No, her pursuer was too close. Her best bet was to reach her car.

Nia increased her speed. She was member of the SUEC volleyball team, and in excellent shape, but her pursuer kept up. There were few people on the promenade—an embracing couple, kissing, not taking notice of their surroundings, and three students at the edge of the promenade, looking for the source of the alarm sirens in the village. As she passed them, Nia shouted, "Fire! Fire!" They turned around and stepped into the middle of the path, looking around.

Nia heard a cursing voice and angry screams. Her pursuer had crashed into them. The footsteps behind her had stopped—for a minute.

Then Nia heard them again. She increased her speed, trying to avoid broken tree branches and pinecones on the dimly lit path. If she tripped, she would be done. Beads of sweat ran down her chest.

The footsteps behind her were catching up. The lower edge of her laptop in her pack hit her back every time her feet impacted the ground. But the laptop could also shield her back. *Don't shoot again!* Nia prayed.

Nia's flank started to hurt. She would not be able to hold this speed for long. She tried to encourage herself. *If they stop to aim at me, they will risk losing me in the darkness.*

Nia saw the parking lot coming closer. Her heart pounded, and she felt dizzy. *Focus!* She reminded herself. *You got this!*

The footsteps behind her seemed to speed up. Her pursuer was closing in.

Nia kept running down the promenade, past the entrance to the parking lot and towards the main entrance gate of the university. She did not want to make her plan too obvious. The parking lot was to the right, separated from her by a wall of rhododendrons. A sweet scent from the opulent flower clusters filled the air.

Nia knew the area by heart. She had taken a short cut from the parking lot through the bushes many times. She heard the footsteps of her pursuer directly behind her. There were no more people on the street.

The footsteps behind her stopped.

But Nia had reached her destination. She jumped into a small gap between two rhododendron bushes as a bullet hit the tree beside her. She cried out in horror, leaped into the parking lot, ran towards her yellow Volkswagen Beetle, grabbed the car key in her pocket, and activated the door opener. Her car greeted her with a *blip, blip* sound and blinking headlights.

Nia jerked the door open, jumped onto the driver's seat, smashed the door shut, pushed the start button, and pressed the gas pedal down to the bottom of the carriage. She heard two high-pitched sounds and breaking glass as she backed out of her spot. She changed the gear, and her car jumped forward, racing down the parking lot.

A cool breeze hit her neck. Nia looked into the mirror and saw that the rear window had burst. The mysterious person was standing in the lot behind her, aiming at her with the gun.

Nia hit the gas harder. The car raced towards the promenade. In front of her, she saw a security guard appearing at the gate, walking into the middle of the gateway, waving at her with raised arms and signaling to stop. She pressed the gas pedal harder, aiming at the gate. The guard jumped out of the way, and the Beetle raced through the gate.

Nia cried out in triumph. She had made it!

She drove down the street that led her to the US-101 highway, away from this horrible place.

***

She arrived in San Francisco about half an hour later. Nobody had followed her. At least, she had not noticed anyone. Her pursuer had worn a motorcycle suit. If they had a bike somewhere, it probably took them some time to get it.

Nia welcomed the sight of the city fog, which lingered like a cool blanket over the city. She hit the gas and dived in. Fluffy clouds embraced her. A perfect cover. Cool air came into the overheated car from the broken rear window, and she inhaled it like a cool drink.

She still heard the gunshots in her head. Terrifying. She tried to focus on the road and reminded herself to calm down. *Stop at the red traffic light. Wait. Green. Continue.* Driving down the street seemed like a mundane task. *What if her pursuer tracked the laptop?*

She tasted bilious acid on her tongue, and her chest tightened. It was difficult to breathe. She felt dizzy, on the verge of a breakdown—physically and mentally. *Focus*, she told herself. She had a good head start.

She reduced her speed as she entered Junipero Serra Boulevard. She took a turn at Portola Drive and then drove up the hill towards Mt. Davidson. Soon, she reached a quiet residential street lined with single-family homes, a mix of Victorian style, Shingle-style and contemporary architecture. The windows of the houses were dark. It was close to midnight. Everyone here was asleep.

Nia stopped in front of a narrow Stick house with a light-yellow façade and white ornamental detailing. The full moon above the house illuminated sunburst-designed rosettes and ornamental truss work at the apex of the gable roof.

Nia got out of her car, walked towards the rustic oaken door, and rang the bell. No response. She rang the doorbell again. A dog inside started barking. She heard the pouring sound of a moving camera above the door. She looked up into the camera and waved. A minute later, the door opened, and Heinz looked at her. His large body filled out most of the doorway. His German Shepherd Schnitzel squeezed himself through a gap between his owner and the doorframe and welcomed Nia with excitement, jumping up and down at her with a rotating tail. Nia leaned down, patted Schnitzel's head and scratched him behind his ears. The dog jumped up and nuzzled her face.

"Nia, what are you doing here in the middle of the night?" Heinz asked.

"I'm sorry, Heinz. I did not know where else to go. I don't have much time to explain. Someone with a gun is chasing me. They shot at me twice. I believe they might want the information about my research on this laptop computer." She pointed at the backpack in her hand. "It's possible that they can track it. Can you please take it and keep it safe?"

Nia reached into her backpack and handed the laptop to Heinz. He looked at her with wide open eyes.

"The password is NiaJ2033."

Heinz shook his head. "Did you ever hear about secure passwords?"

"Sorry—when I set this up, I had no idea that anyone would ever have an interest in my research. The university has an automatic backup system and can track it. You are an IT expert, so I thought you could turn it off."

"Yes, of course I can do that."

"Please be quick. I really don't want to get you in danger, Heinz. I hope it will take them some time to locate the laptop."

"No worries. I can turn it off in an instant. What is so important on it that someone wants to kill you for it?"

"I cannot explain this right now. I have to get out of here as quickly as possible. I will fly home and call you from there."

"Why don't you call the police right now?"

"I'm sorry, but I don't trust the police. SUEC is very powerful, and I don't know who's behind this. Who will the police believe, the SUEC leadership or a black girl?"

Heinz looked at her. "You look awful." He waved at the hallway behind him. "Do you want to come in and at least take a break?"

"No, I want to get as far away as possible. I'll drive to the airport and try to get on the next flight home to Saint Lucia. I will call you from there."

Heinz looked at her. "Okay. Please be careful!"

Nia hugged him. "I am so glad I found you!"

He stroked the back of her head. "Me too! Take care, sister!"

Nia walked back to her car, waved back at Heinz, got in, and closed the door. She leaned back and closed her eyes for just a moment. She was so tired! But she had to pull through.

She started the car and drove towards the Glen Park district. As she approached the ramp to the interstate I280, it became busier again. The headlights of the approaching cars on the other side of the streets were so bright!

Nia squeezed her eyes. *Irritating!* Perhaps these drivers had not turned off their bright lights? All of them? The yellow lines in the middle of the street appeared smudgy. She had difficulty focusing, as if she were drunk or something.

She noted the ramp to the highway too late. The sign to the San Francisco Airport appeared out of nowhere. She hit the brakes and turned left towards the ramp. A car behind her honked and drove around her, the driver flipping a finger at her as she drove up the ramp. There was so much noise here! Several cars rushed by. It was difficult to see the lanes in the darkness of the night.

Another turn to get onto the US-101. Nia slowed down and tried to stay in the right lane. Her eyelids felt so heavy! Was there something on the street? A dead skunk? Nia turned leftwards to drive around it. A car to her left honked wildly, racing by. Nia pulled the car to the right side again. She heard police sirens in the distance. Were the police looking for her?

Nia hit the gas. The car picked up speed. She saw another sign to the airport. Almost there. Dense fog was settling on her windshield. She turned the wipers on. It did not help much. Or was the fog in front of her eyes?

She didn't see the curve in the road. The car raced straight ahead. She saw a tree coming closer and closer, and then, the car crashed into it. The seatbelt kicked in and the airbags deployed. The car stopped.

Nia caught her breath. She moved her arms and her legs. Nothing broken. She felt dizzy. Perhaps a concussion. She looked in the rear mirror. No injuries in her face. Thank God.

There was an approaching motorcycle. She had to get out. She released the seatbelt and pulled on the door handle. The door was stuck. The motorcycle stopped beside her car. Nia started to panic and pushed frantically against the door. The front end of her Beetle was smashed, and the window of the driver's door had crashed to pieces. It would not open. A dark shadow appeared in the window frame. A motorcycle helmet looked at her with cold green eyes.

"Siri," Nia said.

Hm hm, her iPhone responded.

"Green eyes."

There was the high-pitched sound again. Everything was silent at last.

- 4 -

LILI

The Call
Wednesday, May 25, 2033, 1:15 am.

Lili had just gone to bed. The cool temperature of the unused bed turned into a lulling warmth that embraced her body and soothed her busy mind.

Her sleeping self went down a dark tunnel and emerged in a peaceful dream of a warm summer day. She and her husband Mark walked down a sandy beach, hand in hand. Just the two of them. The waves of the ocean roared as they rose and crashed, sending sparkling water onto the shore that embraced their bare feet. A light breeze was gently blowing over the dark blue sea, making her hair flutter. Mark turned around and kissed her.

The musical tone of her phone cut through the serene scene. Real-life Mark, in the bed beside her, cursed. "Spouses of physicians should get paid a premium for interrupted sleep at night!"

"You are a physician as well, Mark."

"Yes, we are double-burdened, and should get a double premium for constant sleep deprivation!" He turned around and pulled the blanket over his head.

Lili got up and walked to her home office. The radiology resident on the phone had a shaky voice. "Hello, Lili, sorry to disturb you. We just received a patient who was dead on arrival. They got a CT scan here for forensic reasons. The ER physicians are asking for a review and final signature by the attending radiologist to finalize our imaging report. There is a large group of people here—policemen, reporters, and spectators."

"Let me have a look at the scan. Can you give me the medical record number or spell the name of the patient?" Lili sat down at her desk and turned on the SUEC workstation.

"N-i-a J-o-h-n-e-s."

"What? This can't be true." Lili typed the name into the system and found a set of new CT images of the woman's head. There was a large hole in the left side of the calvarium, a track of damaged tissue, blood, hair, and bone fragments across the brain, and another hole on the other side of the skull. Large bone fragments had been pushed outwards into the soft tissues of the head.

Lili scrolled through the images in disbelief. "Your report is complete and accurate!" she said. She signed the report to release it to the ER and the electronic medical records.

"Thank you, Dr. Pham," the resident responded. "Actually, the ER physician, Dr. Annya Segond, just walked in, and would like to talk with you as well."

Lili heard a rustling noise as the phone was handed over to Annya. "Hello, Lili, sorry to bother you again. The police could not find Nia in time. She was shot."

"I could glean that from the images. Did they arrest the shooter?"

"No. When the police arrived at the scene, the shooter had already escaped. They are searching for him or her."

"Why was Nia shot? Terrel Wright was with you at her apartment tonight. Is this a matter of national security? Are we all in danger?"

"We do not know yet. Terrel is concerned that it could have to do with Nia's work at SUEC. Infectious-disease research is a hot topic these days."

"What type of infections did she study?"

"Her main area of research was on gender disparities. Nia had a master's degree in genetics and a PhD in infectious diseases from the University College in London, UK. She studied different responses of men and women to infections."

"I cannot imagine someone would kill her for that."

"Perhaps she made a groundbreaking discovery. Something that could make a lot of money."

"I just googled her name, and I did not find any high-impact publication. Nothing in *Nature*, *Science*, the *New England Journal,* or the like. No recent publications at all. No pending patents either."

"Well, the police found more medical imaging studies on the iPhone in her backpack. That's the main reason why I wanted to talk with you. I just sent them to you via a secure email."

"Okay, let me have a look." Lili opened the file.

"Well, this seems to be an easy one. There is a consolidation in the left lower lung. In addition, there is a large pleural effusion. This appears to be a typical bacterial pneumonia. A typical underlying germ would be pneumococcus, but, of course, there are many other bacteria that can create such a picture."

"What about the second file?" Annya asked.

Lili opened it. "Well, this CT scan also shows pneumonia, and it is more severe than the previous case. The patient has a consolidation in both lungs. In addition, there are large cavities within the abnormal lung on the left side. This is a cavitating pneumonia, a pneumonia that formed abscesses. Possible germs are pneumococcus, staphylococcus aureus, and klebsiella, among others."

"So, altogether, we found medical imaging studies of four different patients with four different pneumonias," Annya said.

"Do you see a gender pattern? You said that this was Nia's area of research." Lili said.

"I don't see a pattern yet. Half of the patients here are males, and half are females, but I do believe Nia's assassination must have to do with her work. All SUEC computers have a GPS chip, and according to the GPS tracking system, Nia carried her laptop with her when she left her apartment. But the GPS signal of her computer got lost shortly before she died. Someone must've stolen it."

"But if it had to do with the medical imaging studies on her iPhone, why did the thief not take that as well—or destroy it?" Lili wondered.

"I don't know. Perhaps there wasn't enough time. The police followed the GPS signal of her phone and arrived at the scene literally one minute after she was shot. They saw a motorcycle disappearing in the adjacent forest and pursued it immediately, but they lost it."

"Nia was a postdoctoral researcher, a trainee. If she had made a groundbreaking discovery, wouldn't a killer target her supervisor, her professor?"

"Perhaps. Terrel already called Nia's lab supervisor, Dr. Cristina Maria Walker-Díaz, and ordered a police officer to watch her home. She was completely shocked, understandably."

"Oh, Cristina! I am so sorry! This must be awful for her!" Lili exclaimed.

"Do you know her?" Annya asked.

"She has a lab in the same research building as me, although on a different floor. My imaging lab is on the first floor and her lab is on the second floor. I often see her in the hallway."

"I know her also—she lives in the apartment next to me. But I haven't had much time to talk with her. I'm just always in the clinic. What is she like?"

"She is an Assistant Professor who established her own lab only two years ago. Very nice, very sociable. She always seems to be in a good mood. She greets other researchers in our building and strikes up conversations with total strangers in the cafeteria. That's how I got to know her."

"Well, Terrel will talk with her tomorrow. In the meantime, please keep your eyes open. A SUEC researcher has been killed. There was a shooter at Nia's apartment and a shooter on the highway. We do not know if these were one and the same or two different people. We do not know if they plan to kill more people. And it is very well possible that they are still walking around on campus."

"Don't scare me!"

"I just want you to be careful, Lili. I remember you love to play detective. This is too dangerous for a private investigation."

"Of course! I'll just keep my eyes open and let you know if I see anything unusual. I'm glad that the FBI is helping."

"Yes, the disappearance of the laptop was enough for Terrel to get involved. He is very experienced, and he will find the killer. Thanks for looking at the imaging studies, Lili! See you tomorrow."

"Take care, Annya!"

Lili hung up the phone. She looked again at the imaging studies that Annya had sent her. *How are they connected?*

- 5 -

HEINZ

The Laptop
Wednesday, May 25, 2033, 1:15 am.

Heinz Tremblay walked back into his home with Schnitzel in tow. He took Nia's laptop, stopped in the kitchen to fetch a beer from the fridge, and walked up the stairs to his home office. It was late, but he didn't mind. Working at night filled him with a sense of peacefulness and serenity, and since he lived alone, he could live by his own schedule.

Heinz sat down at his steel-and-wood Ikea desk and opened the laptop. Schnitzel curled up at his feet. Heinz looked through the files on the computer. He found the icon for the backup software and the GPS locator on the upper right side of the task bar.

He opened the beer bottle and a bag of potato chips. The smell of malt, hops, cheese, and onion filled the air. The dog raised his head, licked his lips, and stared at Heinz while the chips crunched between his teeth. Heinz patted Schnitzel's head and focused his attention on the computer screen. He had to delete all traces before anyone could find him.

It only took a few clicks to deactivate the data backup system. Another minute, and the GPS tracking system was out as well. Then, Heinz deleted Nia's files on the backup disk at SUEC and the records of the location of the laptop in the last few hours.

The potato chip bag was almost empty. The dog sat up and placed his paw on Heinz's lap. Heinz looked at him. "Schnitzel, I am busy!"

The dog wagged his tail and responded with a gentle bark. Heinz threw a handful of potato chips on the hardwood floor. They scattered in all directions. Schnitzel grunted approvingly as he chased down the delicious snacks.

Heinz smiled. Schnitzel was his best friend.

He turned his attention back to Nia's computer and opened the folder labeled *Fambly*. It contained an Excel sheet and multiple imaging files, which were labeled as patient 1, 2, 3 etc., up to 22. Heinz opened the excel file. It contained a table, which listed twenty-two patients along with their study number, names, age, gender, race/ethnicity, clinical diagnosis, and dates of two or more imaging studies. This was the patient list.

Heinz searched for his own number. Patient five. It felt weird to be reduced to a number, although Nia had explained to him that this number should protect his privacy. Only she would know the identity of the study subjects. Everyone else would only see a number.

Heinz opened the file of patient five. He read the description in the comment box of the file: *CT scan of the chest shows ground-glass opacities of the lungs bilaterally, predominantly at the lung bases. Importantly, there is no segmental consolidation, no cavitating lesion, and no lymphadenopathy. The findings suggest an atypical pneumonia that is caused by a non-bacterial organism, such as mycoplasma, pneumocystis carinii, or viruses.*

Heinz remembered when he had been diagnosed with COVID-19. It had been scary when he had been alone in his bed with a hundred-degree fever, breathing difficulties, severe headaches, and weakness that made it difficult to walk. He had been so careful, using a facemask every time he went outside, practicing extreme social distancing, ensuring thorough hand hygiene, and doing no travel at all—and then he had caught the virus anyways. Probably somewhere at the grocery store. That was the only place where he'd had contact with other human beings during the pandemic. All other interactions had been via Zoom for months. He sighed. No need to dwell on bad memories. He was fine now.

Heinz tapped on the next file. Patient #6. The comment box stated: *COVID-19 in a 14-year-old girl, patchy airspace consolidation with surrounding ground glass opacities. Note less extensive changes in a child. These findings resolved completely on follow up.*

Another file. Patient #7. The comment box stated: *COVID-19 in a forty-year-old woman, ground glass opacities and interlobular septal thickening, resolved completely on follow up.*

Schnitzel had tracked down all potato chips on the floor and came back for more. Heinz patted him gently. The dog looked at him attentively, licking his lips. Heinz smiled. Schnitzel was always looking for food. His appetite was insatiable. But with Schnitzel at his side, Heinz never felt lonely. And it was impossible to eat alone.

Heinz turned his attention back to the computer screen. It was late, but probably a good idea to create some backups before they retreated for the night. Heinz inserted an ultra-fit drive into the USB port and downloaded all files onto it. He looked around for a secure place where he could hide the tiny device. It was smaller than a coin. Schnitzel noted his wandering gaze and came closer, wagging his tail. Heinz scratched his chin. "Clearly, I have been looking for you," he said to his beloved dog.

Schnitzel looked at Heinz with his large, soulful eyes. He sniffed at the USB drive. Smells were informing his world. He looked disappointed. No food.

Heinz got an idea. Perhaps Schnitzel could help. He opened the upper drawer of his desk and searched around between pens, paperclips, old keys, postcards, post-its, and the like. After a while, he found what he had been looking for: Gorilla glue. He opened the small bottle, added a few drops of glue on the cap of the USB drive, and attached the drive to the lower part of Schnitzel's collar. He held the drive-in place with his left thumb, while scratching Schnitzel in his favorite place behind his right ear. The dog closed his eyes and did not move.

After a few minutes, Heinz checked the device. It was firmly attached to the collar. Heinz looked at the dog. From a distance, it was not possible to see the USB drive, which was covered by Schnitzel's fur. And Schnitzel did not let any strangers get close to him.

Heinz closed the laptop and got up from his large, highbacked desk chair. "Let's call it a night!" he said to the dog. He switched off the lights and walked across the hallway to his bedroom. Schnitzel followed closely and settled on his plush pet bed beside Heinz's bed.

- 6 -

TERREL

The Suspect
Wednesday, May 25, 2033, 8 am.

FBI agent Terrel Wright drove slowly through the gated entrance of SUEC University. The guard at the entrance checked his badge and waved him through the open ornate iron gates. Terrel passed by the tall ornamental limestone columns towards the parking lot. It was a typical California day. The sun already sat high in the spotless dark blue sky, burning away the last streaks of the morning fog.

Terrel parked his car under a large palm tree. Another SUEC guard strolled towards him and asked if he could help him find anything. What the guy really meant to say was that he was out of place here. Terrel showed him his FBI badge. A white woman and two teenagers exited the car next to him and looked at them with suspicion. The women checked twice that the car was locked and rushed the kids towards the other end of the parking lot, where they disappeared behind the trees. The SUEC guard looked at his badge a minute too long, and Terrel wondered if he knew what an authentic FBI badge looked like.

Finally, the guard showed him the path to the University promenade that led to the research buildings. Terrel thanked him, straightened his suit, and moved on.

He felt the constant pressure to justify his existence in the world of the privileged. But he had no regrets. He was aware that he was a trailblazer, an example of black excellence, a role model, and not only at elite colleges, but at his job as well. He had been recently promoted to Deputy Assistant Special Agent in Charge, the second-highest-ranking FBI investigator in Northern California. Many of his colleagues had congratulated him. But there were also others who were jealous and disapproved of a black man in this position. Every day, he did not only have to prove that *he* was capable of doing the job, but he was here to represent his community. Failure was not an option. He had to live up to the expectations.

Terrel was up for the challenge. He was good at his job, and he knew it.

He walked up the flower-lined promenade, following the signs to the research campus. The air tasted of pine trees and lilac, which lined the path to the University village. So sweet. He heard a loud voice behind him say, "On your left!" and stepped aside just in time to let a group of chatting and laughing students pass by on their bicycles. *Nia had been one of them,* he thought.

His own son Niles was still in kindergarten. Would he apply to SUEC one day? Terrel could not bear if anything happened to him. *The poor parents. They probably have been notified by now that their daughter has been murdered.* The most horrifying phone call any parent could possibly imagine.

Terrel felt a shiver running down his spine. He tried to focus on the path in front of him. *I will find the guy who killed her!* he thought as he approached the SUEC village.

He counted about fifteen limestone buildings in the distance, nestled in the green valley of the SUEC campus. Steep, forested hills formed a natural bulwark around the small settlement, as if it were the most secure place in the world. The gate to the SUEC campus was always guarded, and it was difficult to find the way around the University campus in bright daylight, let alone at night. *The murderer must be an insider,* Terrel thought. *The number of suspects will be very limited. I will find him.*

Terrel reached the first buildings and continued to walk along a small park towards the octagonal limestone building in the center of the research campus. Annya had given him the address. Nia had worked here. The building was three stories high with large floor-to-ceiling semi-circular glass windows that shimmered in the morning sun.

Terrel stepped towards the sliding glass doors at the entrance. They did not open. He looked around for a bell but did not find any. Above the door, he noticed a camera, and held his FBI badge towards the sensors.

The voice of a young man emanated from one of the rosebushes besides the door, as if the flowers were speaking. "Hello, Agent Wright. I expected you. I will be there in just a second."

The bush must contain a hidden microphone, Terrel thought. He did not answer. *Too awkward to talk to a rose bush.*

Two minutes later, a young white man in a silver SUEC suit appeared at the other side of the door. He had long blonde hair held together with a hairband in a ponytail. The glass doors opened. "Welcome!" he said with a serious expression on his face. "Please come in!"

Terrel nodded slightly. He looked at the man. Green eyes. "Thank you! Are you Dr. Walker-Díaz?"

The man chuckled. "No, I am Jacub Bezdomny, the building manager. I will bring you to the professor. Please, come this way."

The air inside the building was pleasantly cool. They stepped into the large central atrium, which spanned all three floors of the building and culminated in a stained-glass dome. The incoming sunlight formed a stunning light theater of multicolored rays around them.

"You are the building manager? How long have you been working here?" Terrel asked as they walked through the foyer towards a spiraling central staircase with a double-helix design.

"I got this job three years ago," Jacub answered. "I was in a bad place then. I'd lost my job as a bartender, was evicted from my apartment, and lived in my car for a while. The job offer from SUEC was a turning point for me. They saved my live!"

"Good for you."

The manager looked at him from the corner of his eye. "You are from the FBI. I thought I tell you right away in case you want to check *me* out."

"Should I?"

"I don't think so. I am an honorable man."

"Then you have nothing to worry about.'

They walked up the stairs.

"What attracted you to SUEC?" Terrel asked.

"The receptionist!"

Terrel laughed.

They reached the second floor and walked down a long, white-walled hallway. It smelled of chlorine bleach. To the right, they passed multiple entrances to science labs where young people in white coats were sitting at benches covered with laboratory glassware and electrical devices, stirring chemicals into Erlenmeyer flasks, holding test tubes over Bunsen burners, or ambulating smoldering materials in fume hoods.

"So, Nia was shot last night?" Jacub asked with another quick look at Terrel.

"Yes, indeed."

"Do you know who did it?"

"Not yet. But I am here to find out."

They had arrived at an opaque glass office door with Dr. Cristina Walker-Díaz's name on it. Jacub hesitated for a moment. "Be nice to her, man. She has the most integrity of any person I know on this campus."

"I thought that was you?"

"You know what I mean."

"No worries. I'm just looking for some information," Terrel responded.

Jacub knocked at the door. They heard a melodic voice from inside. "Please come in!"

Jacub opened the door. "Hello, professor. FBI agent Terrel Wright is here to see you."

Terrel gleaned over Jacub's shoulder and saw an exceptionally attractive woman with perfectly coiffed hair behind an oversized oak desk. "Thank you, Jacub!" Dr. Díaz said with a soft voice. "Agent Wright, please come in."

Terrel stepped into the small office and looked around as Jacub turned and shut the door behind him. The large desk occupied most of the room. On the wall behind Dr. Díaz were framed group photos of her surrounded by smiling young people, perhaps her research team. Terrel recognized Nia. She looked happy.

Terrel cleared his throat. "I am so sorry for the loss of your team member," he said.

Cristina Walker-Díaz dabbed her lower eyelids with a paper towel. "I still cannot understand what happened. Nia was shot! This is so horrible. Would you like to sit?" She pointed at a chair in front of the desk.

Terrel sat down. He noticed smudged mascara around her hazel eyes and watery dark lines running down her cheeks. Around her neck was a necklace with a large golden ornamental cross. "Dr. Díaz, I understand that this is a very traumatic situation. I am here to find the person who is responsible for this crime. Would you be able to answer a few questions?"

He tried to establish eye contact, but Dr. Díaz focused on her tissue paper. Her hands trembled. "Of course," she whispered.

Terrel fetched his notebook. "Again, I'm so sorry for your loss. Have you been very close with Nia?"

"Well, I have a small team. Nia was one of three postdoctoral fellows in my lab."

"How long has Nia been working with you?"

"A little over two years. She came highly acclaimed, with a master's degree in genetics and a PhD in infectious diseases from the University College in London."

"And your lab studies infectious diseases as well?"

"Yeah, our team studies the role that genes play in our ability to fight infections. For example, we study differences between sexes. In many instances, women mount stronger immune responses compared to men. There are, of course, many nuances here, but in general, many females clear pathogens faster than males. This stronger immune response can also lead to problems. For example, 80% of autoimmune diseases occur in females."

Her pale cheeks flushed slightly as she talked about her research, but she still evaded Terrel's probing gaze. Was she hiding something?

"And what was Nia's project?" he asked.

"She was supposed to study long-term clinical problems after a COVID-19 infection. Despite the higher mortality in men, women tend to be at higher risk for long-term COVID-19 complications. We have a large database of COVID survivors, and Nia was supposed to analyze their data with regards to sex differences."

"You said twice that she was *supposed* to study this. Are you implying that this was the plan, but she did not do it?"

"Correct." Cristina kept looking at her tissue paper, folding it around in her hands.

"What did she do instead?"

"She collected medical imaging studies from a wide range of infectious diseases. We do not really do that in my lab."

"She did not follow your instructions?"

"Exactly. Every trainee in my lab focuses on a specific gene or genetic trait that encodes the sensitivity to a specific pathogen. That then allows us to issue recommendations for disease prevention and develop personalized therapies. But Nia would not listen. She would study viral infections today, tuberculosis tomorrow, and fungal infections after that. You cannot draw any scientific conclusions from such an unfocused approach."

"I see. And that made you angry?"

Cristina now looked at him. "You bet! The National Institute of Health paid Nia's salary for investigating long COVID. She did not produce anything. How should I write a progress report for the NIH? How should I get more research funding? How should we make progress if our team members just ignore their work assignments?"

"I understand. Did you confront her about your concern?"

"I sure did! She told me that she was working on COVID infections. She lied!" Cristina flipped through a pile of papers on her desk. She fetched a printout of a CT scan and held it in front of Terrel. "See this!"

Terrel looked at the CT scan. "What does it show?" he asked.

"This image shows of a large thrombus in the right and left pulmonary artery of a child with COVID-19 infection. The thrombus is occlusive. That means it fills out the entire vessel. That impairs the perfusion of the lung and the oxygenation of the blood. The thrombus extends into some of the branches of the pulmonary artery. Such an extensive thrombus can be fatal if left untreated." Cristina pointed at the abnormalities.

"So, Nia *did* work on COVID?"

"Well, a few of the imaging studies that she collected showed a COVID infection. But most of the others showed other infections. In addition, this patient here was treated with an extraction of the thrombus and recovered completely. They did not develop long COVID, the condition that Nia was supposed to study."

"Do you know why she collected these images?"

"I once was so upset about her lack of progress that I looked through the patient list on her desk. I do not usually micromanage, but this was a special situation. I just wanted to understand what she was up to. To my surprise, I saw that all patients on her list had a history of in vitro fertilization. That made me even more angry!"

"Why would that make you angry?"

"Everyone knows that patients who were conceived by IVF have a higher risk of developing a wide range of illnesses, including infections. There's nothing new to study there. And I certainly don't want to spend my research dollars on it." She clutched her left hand around the cross on her chest and raised her right index finger. "Humans should not play god! How can anyone be so audacious to think they can decide which embryo will live or die?"

"You have moral reservations against IVF practices?" Terrel asked. He made a note in his notebook.

Cristina nodded. "Yes, sir. I have moral and technical concerns. Even if we can unite an egg and sperm in a test tube, this does not mean that we are authorized or capable of doing it. For example, how would we get a soul in whatever we created?"

Terrel shrugged. "I don't know. I have a niece who was conceived by IVF, and I would say that she is very soulful, whatever that means."

"Yeah, you can be lucky. All I'm saying is that we think we know how to make humans, when in fact we only know how to make the shell. Some eggs and sperms were not meant to be together. God might decide not to add a soul."

Terrel nodded as if he understood. "So, it was against your moral beliefs that Nia investigated infections in patients conceived by IVF?"

"I told her to stop. And she would not *listen*!" Cristina's eyes tightened, and sparks of fire seemed to dart at Terrel.

"Did you threaten to fire her?" he asked. It was a best guess, considering all that had been said.

Cristina nodded slowly, looking at the desk in front of her. "I am sorry I did. I feel bad about it now."

"Dr. Díaz, I am very sorry for these unfortunate events, and I understand your concerns. I'm wondering if Nia's personal project has something to do with her death. Do you know if she collaborated with anyone on this? Can you imagine anyone who might want to harm her?"

"I don't know. Apart from the fact that she did not focus on her project, she was very pleasant to work with. I did not ever see her arguing with anyone. Even with me, she was always very composed. I never knew what was going on in her head."

"Thank you for sharing this information with me." Terrel looked at Cristina, who wiped her eyes with a Kleenex. "Do you need a break?"

"Well, what should I say? My student was shot. I don't think I will feel better anytime soon. What else do you need to know?"

"I have to ask you one more question: Where were you last night between ten p.m. and two a.m.?"

Cristina looked at him with raised eyebrows. "Am I a suspect now?"

"This is a routine question. I can assure you that I have to ask this of everyone I interview."

"Well, I was in my bed."

"Do you have a witness?"

"That I was sleeping? I am afraid I was alone."

"Where do you live?"

"I live in the faculty housing apartment complex on Redwood Avenue, here in the SUEC valley."

"Is that the same building where Nia lived?"

"No, it's about half a mile away."

"Thank you." Terrel closed his notebook and got up from his seat. "This was very helpful. If you can think of anything else that might help us finding the shooter, please call me." He pulled a business card from his pocket and handed it to Cristina.

"Of course, I will!" Her gaze went past him to the door.

Terrel turned around. He opened the office door and almost ran into Jacub, who was standing on the other side, exactly where he had left him.

"Oh! Did you wait here the whole time?" Terrel asked, while thinking, *Was he eavesdropping?*

"Hello, Agent Wright." Jacub flashed two rows of perfectly white teeth. "No. I ran some errands and just came back. Looks like this was perfect timing. Should I lead you back to the entrance? It can be difficult to find your way around here."

"That's kind of you," Terrel said. He looked at Jacub. Did he want to prevent him from looking around?

Jacub returned an innocent smile. "Come this way, please."

They walked back to the atrium. Terrel felt the sun above him penetrating the multicolored glass cupola. Rays of rainbow colors embraced him and Jacub as they descended the stairs.

"Did you know Nia?" Terrel asked.

"Of course. She works here," Jacub responded.

"When did you see her the last time?"

"Yesterday afternoon."

"Is that right? When and where was that?"

"Here in the building, around six p.m., I guess."

"Did you notice anything unusual about her?"

"Well, she sent me an email to pick up toothpaste for her at the grocery store next door. I sometimes run errands for our tenants here, you know. Gives me a little extra income."

"And that request was unusual?"

"Yeah, when I brought her the toothpaste, she seemed to have forgotten about it. I told her not to worry. I could just keep it for myself. Then she took it."

"Hm. That is interesting, indeed. Did you buy toothpaste for her before?"

"No, not for her. Most of the time, I run errands for our faculty. They tip generously. So, it's a great side gig. But postdoctoral fellows are usually short on cash and would rather run to the shop by themselves."

"So, this was unusual?"

"Yeah, I guess, although I do sometimes get a request from one of the trainees, mostly when they're close to an exam or some other deadline and are stressed out. So, I didn't think too much about it."

"I see. Was Nia close to an exam or deadline?"

"I don't know. The people in the building here rarely share that much detail with me."

"Can you think of anyone who might want to hurt her?"

"No, not really. I didn't know her that well, but I liked her. There are a lot of entitled people around here, people who have never said a single word to me. Nia was genuinely friendly, and she never made me feel like I was beneath her. She always smiled and greeted me. She opened doors for strangers and let people cut in front of her in the coffee line. She treated everyone with *respect*." Jacub's voice had raised slightly.

Terrel made a mental note. Respect was very important to him, as it was for many minority members who encountered discrimination and oppression on a regular basis.

They had reached the entrance of the building. Terrel shook Jacub's hand. "Thank you, Mr. Bezdomny."

He smiled. "Any time!"

Terrel walked out of the building. This time, he watched Jacub walking away through the glass door.

Then he pulled his cell phone and called his forensic team. "Hi, this is Terrel. When you go to Nia Johnes' apartment today, can you please do a tox screen of her toothpaste?"

- 7 -

JACUB

The Attack
Wednesday, May 25, 2033, 8:30 am.

Jacub walked back to his office. Time for a break.

His office faced the east side of the building, and the air in the room had been heated by the California sun. He did not like to turn up the air conditioner. It dried up the room and made his eyes feel itchy. He went to the large window in the back of the room and opened it. A cool breeze entered the room, tinted with the fragrance of the eucalyptus trees and rhododendron bushes that separated the research building from a small nearby park.

Jacub inhaled deeply and turned to the refrigerator behind his desk. He fetched a smoked kielbasa sausage, bread, mustard, and kvass. He licked his lips, then sat down on the convertible sleeper sofa and started eating. The sausage tasted of smoked ham, garlic, cloves, and marjoram. He poured kvass into a glass, leaned back, slipped out of his shoes, and placed his feet on the coffee table in front of him. He took a sip. Life at SUEC was good!

The facetime app on his iPad rang. He sighed and positioned the iPad on his lap so that the video displayed his face. "Hi, mom."

"Jacub, I haven't heard from you for several days! One more day, and I would have reported a missing person!"

"Sorry, mom. I was busy."

"I see you sitting on your couch. Are you lazy?"

"I'm never lazy. I'm on energy-saving mode right now. One of the researchers here was shot last night, and the FBI is investigating the case. I just talked with one of them. I guess this will become a busy week."

"Yes, I heard about the girl on the news this morning. That's why I wanted to make sure you're okay."

"No worries, I'm fine."

"The reporter said that the girl worked in the lab of Dr. Walker-Díaz. I remember that name—you mentioned that she is a researcher in your building. Her student was shot! You could be next!"

"Mom, I'm just the building manager. I'm far too unimportant to be shot by anyone."

"You have always been too trustful, Jacub. Remember when your girlfriend cancelled the lease for your apartment, and you ended up on the street?"

"Ex-girlfriend. And it was her apartment."

"Well, did you learn from that and get your own apartment?"

"For now, I am living in my office here at SUEC. Great room. No commute. No rent. It's perfect."

"Well, what if your boss finds out that you're living in your office?"

"Nobody knows, and nobody cares. We talked about this before. I was told that the SUEC apartments were for faculty and students only, so I arranged my own accommodation. Nobody noticed. And if they do see me here in the evenings, I can just tell them that I had to work late and stayed overnight in my office. Nobody will ever think that I live here."

"The girl was shot at night. You could accidentally get into a shooting scene. I'm afraid you will get hurt!"

"Nia wasn't shot on campus, but on the 101 highway, close to San Francisco. We are in Redwood city here. The SUEC campus is heavily guarded. This is probably the safest place for me to be right now. And imagine how much money I save every month. Together with the errands that I run for the tenants in this building, I save about $6,000 every month. That is $72,000 every year and will be $720,000 in ten years. With that, I can buy a really nice home, and will never have to worry about being kicked out of a rented apartment again."

"You can't really think that you will live there for ten years."

"Why not? It worked out fine so far. Great food in the cafeteria, no noisy neighbors, and a park in the backyard."

"You do not have a bathroom!"

"The bathrooms are right next to my office, and I can shower in the gym next door anytime I want. Plus, I get regular exercise, and I have my own personal swimming pool!" Jacub chuckled.

His mother looked at him, shaking her head. "I wish you had not gone to America. Nothing good has come from it."

"It is only for a while. I will earn some good money here, and then I will retire back home in Poland. With my savings, I can buy a villa for us."

"I hope we will both be alive to see that happen!"

They stayed silent for a moment. Jacob wondered how he could change the subject.

All of a sudden, his mother started screaming. "Jacub, get to the ground! Get down! I see a gun behind you!" Then, she shouted, "You are on camera! I see you! I see you!"

Jacub dropped his plate. He jumped up from the couch and turned around.

There was no one.

"Mom, don't scare me like that!" he complained.

"I saw a gun pointed at your back!" his mother insisted.

Jacub looked at the half-open window again. Was there a rustling noise and movement of the rhododendron bushes on the other side? He stepped towards the window.

"Jacub, get away from that window!" his mother screamed.

Jacub saw a little squirrel climbing up the eucalyptus tree beside the bushes. He turned around. "It was just a squirrel," he said.

"No, it was the barrel of a gun, and it was pointing at your back!" his mother responded. "I saw it very clearly. You must get out of there, Jacub! You are in danger!"

"Mom, it was just a squirrel. Nobody has any reason to shoot me. I will be careful, I promise."

***

The shadow behind the tree waited until Jacub had ended the conversation with his mother. But then he turned around and left the room.

The shadow retreated. There would be another occasion.

- 8 -

LILI

The Secret
Wednesday, May 25, 2033, 9 am.

Lili stopped at the Starbucks coffee booth to the right of the octagonal research building. She yearned for caffeine after her busy night shift. She loved her job, but she also felt drained. The night calls were getting more stressful as she got older. Her legs felt heavy, and her eyes were puffy.

When she was younger, Lili had argued with hospital leadership that attendings on night call should have time off the next day. But her requests had been denied over and over again. The argument of the other side was that she was *only* called for urgent cases. She could get some sleep in between. In the past, she had tried to explain that the adrenaline rush kept her awake long after the case was done. She wished these administrators could join her for just one week of 24/7 calls. *They* should try to sleep after reviewing a scan of a victim of a car crash or a shooting accident.

And what good was two to three hours of sleep anyways? There were minimum hours of uninterrupted rest for truck drivers and pilots. But not for physicians.

By now, she had given up the battle. No point in wasting time with discussions where the other side was determined not to understand. Physicians were in short demand, but, in the absence of physician unions, the administration stretched their workforce as they pleased.

Lili did love her job, and she didn't want to quit over some lost sleep. So, a coffee it was.

The coffee booth was situated at the edge of a park area with a small pond and surrounding flowers, grass, and benches. Lili got into a small line in front of the booth. The air was filled with the fragrance of coffee and fresh baked goods. Lili closed her eyes for just a moment, tuning out the noise from people around her. A slight breeze brushed her face, and the sun embraced her aching spine. To her left, Lili heard chattering ducks and splashing water.

Somebody tapped her shoulder: "Hey, Lili, are you sleeping upright?"

She opened her eyes and saw Cristina Walker-Díaz joining the line behind her. "Hello, Cristina, how are you?"

"Well, thanks for asking. Today is the worst day of my life!"

"I heard about your student. I'm so sorry!"

"I still cannot believe that Nia is dead. The poor parents. I met them a few months ago when they were visiting, and Nia showed them around. They were so proud that their daughter was working at SUEC. The most famous university in the world."

"Yes, this is terrible. I cannot imagine how devastated they must be. Will they fly in from the UK?"

"Nia studied in London, but her parents live in St. Lucia. You know, the Caribbean Island. When they heard about their daughter's death tonight, they booked the next flight here. They will arrive later this morning and meet with Dean Hill. He just called me and asked me to join. But I'm not sure I can." Teers welled up in Cristina's eyes.

"I'm so sorry for your loss." Lili put an arm around her. "*You* have to process Nia's death as well, don't forget that."

Cristina stepped closer and lowered her voice. "I wish I had listened to her more. Just yesterday, we were arguing about her lack of progress with her research project. She wanted to show me some medical images, but I refused to look at them."

"What images?"

"I don't know. She left them on my desk. I flipped through them, but I'm not sure what I was looking at. Would you have a look?"

"Sure, but if they're connected to Nia's death, then you have to hand them over to the police."

"Of course! I would just like to know what they're about first."

They had reached the front of the line. Lili ordered a café latte, and Cristina ordered a black coffee with lots of sugar. They added lids to their cups and strolled through the park. The pond in the middle was lined with rocks and sea lilies. Large freckled goldfish were swimming around, some poking up to the surface, taking flies off the surface, and diving back into the water. A lizard escaped from their approaching feet as they slowly walked towards the research building.

Cristina continued the conversation. "Actually, an FBI agent just visited me. I wanted to show him the images, but he treated me like a suspect, and I didn't want to say anything that would make me look suspicious. I'm mortified by the idea that reviewing the images yesterday could have saved her."

"There's only one way to find out. Let's have a look!"

They had reached the research building, and walked through the large atrium, then up the stairs to the second floor and Cristina's office.

Lili noticed footsteps behind them. She turned around and saw a shadow disappearing in the lab next door.

Was somebody stalking them?

They went into Cristina's office, and Lili closed the door carefully. Cristina flipped through a pile of papers on her desk and pulled out several printouts of imaging studies. "Here they are." She handed them to Lili.

Lili observed the images carefully. "Well, the first one here is a CT scan of the chest with an infiltrate of the left upper lung and multiple calcified lymph nodes. In addition, a CT scan of the neck shows multiple lymph nodes which are centrally necrotic." Lili pointed to the abnormality.

"What about these?" Cristina handed her another set of images. "They have the same case number, number nine, so they are presumably from the same patient."

Lili observed them closely. "These are MRI scans of the head. The first two images of this patient are contrast-enhanced MRIs, which show two ring-enhancing lesions in the cerebellum." Lili pointed at the lesions. "The next two are diffusion weighted images (DWI). The lesions have low signal on the DWI scan. This is helpful in distinguishing them from an abscess."

"What disease do you think this is?" Cristina asked.

"Well, it is almost certainly an infectious disease. Radiologists often cannot pinpoint to one single underlying germ. But taken together, the imaging findings seem to be characteristic for tuberculosis. A lung infiltrate, calcified lymph nodes, necrotic lymph nodes, and what looks like tuberculomas in the brain. As you know, in the clinical setting, this imaging diagnosis would have to be confirmed by lab assays.”

“Of course. I understand. Likely, tuberculosis of the chest and brain.” Cristina made a note.

“Can you have a look at the other images as well?” Cristina handed her prints with the hand-written label *Case Ten*.

“Of course.” Lili looked at the next set of magnetic resonance imaging studies. “These are MR images of a young child. As you can see, there is marked thickening and contrast enhancement along the meninges, most pronounced along the base of the brain. I believe this is another case of tuberculosis. The contrast enhancement along the base of the brain in patients with Tb infection is different to bacterial infections, which typically involve meninges over the brain surfaces.”

Cristina studied the images carefully and made another note in her notebook. “So, two patients with tuberculosis of the brain,” she summarized. “What do the next images show?”

Lili flipped through the next folder. “This is another example of severe meningitis with associated intracerebral lesions,” she said. “Again, the meninges at the skull base are more affected than the meninges over the cerebral hemispheres. Perhaps another case of tuberculosis.”

Cristina turned the images around. “This one has a case number, number eleven, and also a name on it: Ingrid Maulvi.”

“Hm, that name sounds familiar.” Lili tried to remember where she had heard it before.

Cristina looked at her. “Dr. Robinson has a lab manager with the same name.”

“Do you mean Dr. Oliver Stuart Robinson?”

“Yes, that’s him. His lab is right next to mine.”

“Then it should be easy to find her. Let’s go over there and ask her if these are her images.” Lili said.

“Well, I am not exactly on good terms with Dr. Robinson.”

“Is that so? Why not?”

“Well, Dr. Robinson studies *in vitro* fertilization, and he performs pre-implantation diagnoses. That means he investigates fertilized human eggs and decides which ones are to live or not. You might remember, I am a Catholic. My church denounces all forms of assisted reproduction. I cannot approve his actions.”

"Dr. Robinson is also the Vice Dean of Academic Affairs, right? Any promotion at SUEC—including yours—would go through him? Isn't that motivation enough to stay on friendly terms?"

"I am as friendly as possible. But when he starts glorifying IVF, I have to speak up. Children are a gift from God. Nobody should interfere with their conception. Even if science makes manipulation of gametes possible, it does not make it right. I cannot approve what he is doing, and it is best if I just stay out of his way."

Lili cleared her throat. "Okay, I get it. I will stop by his lab and see if I can talk with Ingrid. She might have information that could help us understand what these images mean."

Cristina nodded. "Thank you, Lili! I appreciate it. Indeed, Nia had a patient list on her desk that showed that all of her patients were conceived by IVF. I was really upset when I saw that. Not only was she lacking progress with her assigned project, but she also used my research money to study IVF!"

"Can I see that list?"

"I already looked for it, but it seems that it has disappeared."

"Really? That sounds very suspicious. Did you inform the police about that?"

"Not yet. I don't want to get anyone in trouble here. What if they close my lab down? Perhaps this list is entirely unrelated."

"We clearly need to speak with someone from Dr. Robinson's lab. Perhaps they know more."

"I agree. But considering our debates about IVF in the past, I don't think they would give me any information about a patient list."

"No problem. I will talk with them."

Cristina's eyes filled with tears again. "Thank you, Lili! You are a real friend!"

Lili embraced her. "Feel free to give me a ring any time."

Cristina streaked the corner of her right eye with the back of her hand. "Before you go: There's one more case here. Can you please have a look? This one is labeled as *Control Number 1.*"

Lili looked at another set of images. "Looks like another case of tuberculosis," she said. "Although there is one thing different here: This case includes MR imaging studies from two different time points. The first two images show meningeal contrast enhancement around the cerebellum and pons, as we also observed for the other cases. The second set of images shows marked progression in size and number of the lesions. This patient's infection progressed."

Lili looked at Cristina. "*Control Group* means that there is also a study group. Perhaps the mystery around the images was not in the type of disease, or even the fact that all patients had a history of IVF. Perhaps that's just how she found patients with infections. Perhaps she had a cure?"

Cristina shook her head. "I doubt that she synthesized a new drug. Our lab is relatively small, so if she had done some chemistry here, I would have seen her working on it. And I would have seen bills for chemicals. None of this was the case."

Lili thought about it for a moment. "Yesterday, Annya Segond asked me to look up another set of images that she found in Nia's apartment. That was a pneumonia, and I noted that it resolved completely. So, if we want to find out if this is a pattern for all of these patients, then we need to find the follow-up studies for all of them."

"Or we need to find the drug that she studied. I will look around the lab and check her computer files to see if I can find anything."

"And if Ingrid did have an infection, I will ask her how she was treated." Lili turned around, opened the door, and almost ran into Jacub, the building manager.

"*Ojej!*" he exclaimed.

Both women looked at him. Had he been standing behind the door?

Jacub pointed at a six pack under his arm. "I heard about Nia's death and brought some Inca Kola for Cristina." He looked at her. "I wanted to make you feel a little better. I know you don't eat in times of crisis. But you love these." He pointed at the glass bottles. "And you need to stay hydrated. I ran to the grocery store next door and got some for you."

Cristina's eyes glistened.

"I'm so sorry for your loss!" he added.

"Thank you, Jacub. You are a real friend!" She took a twenty-dollar bill out of her purse and handed it to him. Jacub smiled at both women and left.

Lili waited until she saw a silhouette disappearing down the stairs. Then she said, "Looks like he has a pretty profitable side hustle going on."

Cristina placed the Inca Kola on her desk, "Well, I'm sure a building manager does not earn a fortune. Jacub has a very keen eye, and he knows everyone in the building well. I think it is great that we can contact him to run some errands for us. And, sometimes, he foresees our needs even before we realize them. As far as I'm concerned, I think this is one of his best qualities."

Lili shrugged. "Okay. Whatever works for you. I will see what I can find out next door and will let you know."

- 9 -

TERREL

The Ultimatum
Wednesday, May 25, 2033, 9 am.

FBI agent Terrel Wright walked up the Redwood-lined promenade towards the main administrative building of the university. It was time for a talk with university leadership. The path up the hill was quite steep. The founders of SUEC had deepened the valley and elevated the surrounding mountains to create a private enclosure. But Terrel was physically fit and could easily keep up with the students who walked up the hill beside him. On the serpentinite hilltop, he saw the octagonal university building, which sat like a landed spaceship on the highest mountain in the area. The steel-and-limestone building on the top of the hill was about fifteen meters tall, with multicolored arched windows and a cathedral-like cupola. It was a giant copy of the research building that he had visited earlier this morning. An enormous pedestal and an array of steel columns anchored it on the ground.

Terrel continued the path up the promenade towards the SUEC flagship. Below him, in the valley, the SUEC research building, the lecture hall, library and apartment buildings looked like little offspring of the main octagon in front of him. A group of students stood at the edge of the path and took photos, chatting and laughing. Terrel imagined Nia standing among them. A student at the most famous university of the world. Her parents must have been so proud of her. Now, she was dead. Murdered. What was so precious here that someone would kill her for it? Would the shooter strike again? Was the entire University in danger?

Hopefully, the Dean would have some answers to these questions.

Terrel reached a terrace on the top of the hill, which led to the entrance of the administrative building. To his right was dense forest with majestic Redwoods, Sequoias, and pines. In front of him was a small café where people were drinking their coffee under the shade of the trees. The smell of coffee and cocoa filled the air. Terrel had been up for most of the night, and he craved some caffeine, but he did not want to lose a minute. Perhaps he could grab a cappuccino on his way back. To his right, a raven snatched a half-eaten croissant from a deserted table, taking off high into the air with its prey. Another raven followed with a gurgling croak.

Terrel passed the café and stepped towards the entrance of the octagonal administrative building. He opened the massive double entrance doors and entered the foyer. A breeze of cool air embraced him. He had been looking forward to seeing the Dean's assistant, Aiko, who had helped him capturing a suspect last year, again. But Aiko was not here today. A security guard was sitting at the large, C-shaped entrance desk and helped him to check in. Terrel provided his ID card and stared into the iris detector. A beep signaled that the computer had cleared him. He stepped through the metal detector and walked through the diamond-shaped atrium. In the center of the atrium was a gigantic steel column that rose three stories high and merged into multiple branches, which supported a large multi-colored glass cupola. A matching glass spiral stairway led around the central column to the second floor, where the administrative offices were located.

Terrel walked up the stairs and down a pillared barrel-vaulted hallway until he reached the office of the University Dean, Dr. Robert Hill. He knocked. The door opened right away, and Dr. Hill was standing right in front of him. He must have been on his way out. He looked at Terrel with watery light brown eyes. *Not green*, Terrel thought. He knew Dr. Hill as an honest man of integrity, although, yes, he could not exclude anyone from his investigation because of his status or because he liked him.

"Hello, Agent Wright," Dr. Hill said with a trembling voice. "This is perfect timing. We just finished our meeting." He waved Terrel in.

Terrel stepped into the room and noticed an elderly couple behind Dr. Hill. "These are Mr. and Mrs. Johnes," Dr. Hill said. He turned to the couple. "Mr. and Mrs. Johnes, this is FBI Special Agent Terrel Wright. He is here to find the person who killed your daughter."

Nia's mother looked at Terrel, tears streaming down her cheeks. She wiped her nose with the back of her hand. The despair in her eyes was in stark contrast to the sweet aura of magnolia perfume around her. The man beside her stared at Terrel with a desolate gaze. His face was ash-gray. He groped for the door frame to steady himself.

Mrs. Johnes looked at Terrel. "Where were the police when Nia was shot on the highway? We heard that crime is out of control in San Francisco. But we did not know that students are shot on the streets." Her voice cracked.

Terrel cleared his throat. "I am so sorry for your loss, Mrs. Johnes. As you might've heard, someone shot at Nia in her apartment last night, and she ran away. The police tracked her phone and followed her, but unfortunately, they found her too late."

"If we had only known that she was in trouble," Mrs. Johnes sobbed, wiping her face again with the drenched Kleenex. "If anyone had told us, we would have been able to help her."

"I'm so sorry, Mrs. Johnes. I don't think any of us knew that Nia was in trouble," Terrel responded. He looked from Dean Hill to the parents. Was it the right time to ask his questions? The parents were devastated. But time was of the essence. "Mr. and Mrs. Johnes, do you have any idea who might have harmed your daughter?"

"We thought she was doing well here," Mrs. Johnes responded. "Nia was so excited about being at SUEC. We were all so proud of her. We do not have any doctors in our family, you know. She was the first. She was smart, kind, and generous. She did not have any enemies."

Mr. Johnes cleared his throat. "Well, someone shot Nia, so she had at least one."

Mrs. Johnes looked at him. "Honey, perhaps it was a deadly mistake. Perhaps the shooter thought she was somebody else."

Mr. Johnes shook his head. "I don't know. The murderer came to *her* apartment, he followed *her* car, and he must have looked at *her* when he shot her in the head. That doesn't sound like a mix-up to me at all."

"This is so horrible!" Mrs. Johnes sobbed. Her husband embraced her. He looked exhausted.

Terrel felt a crushing weight on his chest. "Would you like to sit down?" He pointed at seats at the conference table.

"No, we don't," Mr. Johnes responded harshly. "Dr. Hill provided us with all the information we need for now. Perhaps he can fill you in. We told him everything we know."

Dean Hill slightly bowed towards them. "I will discuss the next steps with Agent Wright and keep you updated as soon as we know more. I assure you that we will bring this person to justice."

Mr. Johnes nodded. He looked at Terrel. "So, you have no clue who shot my daughter?"

"My team is collecting the evidence as we speak," Terrel responded. "Did you notice anything unusual? Anything at all that could help us understand what was going on?"

Mrs. Johnes looked up. "Well, a few weeks ago, Nia mentioned that she found her brother, which seemed very odd to me. She's our only child, and I am pretty sure she did not have a brother. I'm her mother."

"Do you know who that brother was?"

"She mentioned a German name," Nia's father responded, "but I do not remember it."

Mrs. Johnes added, "She said that he lived in a beautiful house in San Francisco. She visited him several times, and I was hoping that he was a love interest."

"Nia did not have a boyfriend," Mr. Johnes added, gently stroking his wife's back.

Mrs. Johnes looked at her husband. "I was getting concerned that Nia would never get married. She was so absorbed with her research. I prayed every night that she would meet a nice young man."

"Can you please try to remember his name?" Terrel asked. "This could be important for our investigation. Even if he has nothing to do with the shooting, he might know something."

Mrs. Johnes shrugged. "I'm sorry, that's all we know," Mr. Johnes responded.

There was a moment of silence.

"When can we see her?" Mrs. Johnes asked.

"Your daughter is being examined by a forensic team right now," Terrel explained. "They will complete their work as quickly as possible. As soon as they are done, they will assist you in transferring Nia to St. Lucia. That's where you want her body to go, right?"

Mrs. Johnes nodded slowly, wiping her eyes. "Do you have a daughter?" she asked.

"I have a little son," Terrel responded.

"When you see him tonight, will you hug him for me?"

Terrel swallowed. "I will," he said softly.

"Hug him closely. You'll never know when it will be the last time you see him."

Terrel nodded. The knot in his throat tightened. He did not know what to say.

Mrs. Johnes reached for her husband's hand. "Let's go."

They slowly stepped out, not looking back. The door shut.

Terrel looked at Dean Hill, who looked exhausted as well. "Should we sit down?" he asked.

Robert Hill nodded and pointed to the left. There was a large desk with an oversized swiveling armchair that faced the window and the beautiful view over the valley. To the left of the armchair was a coffee table and a mirroring second armchair. Turning the desk chair around created a nice sitting arrangement for two people. They both sat.

"I am sorry for these unfortunate circumstances," Terrel said. "But I am pleased to meet you here as the new dean. Congratulations!"

"Thank you!" Dr. Robert Hill looked at him. "I was really excited that our board chose me as their dean. The first few months of my appointment have been very fulfilling. We've started several first-in-the-world research initiatives, and we've welcomed a new class of bright, enthusiastic students. We filed multiple new patents, started new industry collaborations, and attracted major donors. We had such a great phase of optimism, innovation, and prosperity. But then hell broke loose. A shooter on campus. A student murdered. And talking with Mr. and Mrs. Johnes was the worst task of my life."

"I can imagine that," Terrel said.

The dean nodded. "I feel so sorry for them. And I continue to wonder if the university could've done anything to prevent this tragedy."

"We already have a strong presence on campus," Terrel responded. "But perhaps we need even more security coverage at a university like this."

"Last time, you came with a colleague?" Robert asked.

"Yeah. This is not an official FBI case yet. I'm here to find out if this case threatens our national security. If it does, then my boss, Angus Weber, will get involved as well. If not, then the police will handle it."

"I understand."

"Either way, Dr. Annya Segond will be a great resource for us. As a physician at SUEC hospital and ex-CIA agent, she can help us make progress in this case."

The dean nodded. "Yes, indeed. I will make sure she will be released from her clinical responsibilities so she can assist you."

"She's helped already. The security team asked her to check on Nia last night, since she lives close by. Unfortunately, Nia had already left when Annya arrived at her apartment. I met her there, and we found medical imaging studies of lung infections on Nia's desk. I was wondering if Nia was working on any high-end research project. Did she have access to sensitive information? Anything that could get her killed?"

"Nia's faculty supervisor, Dr. Cristina Walker-Díaz, is developing new drugs for treating infectious diseases. Pretty powerful stuff. I just learned today that Nia's task was to investigate how men and women respond differently to these new therapies. This should then help to create personalized therapies that are more effective and have fewer side effects than 'one size fits all' treatments. But apparently, Nia wasn't making much progress. I'm not aware of any recent discovery that would be worth killing for."

"I saw Dr. Díaz this morning. She seemed a bit intense."

"Well, she's not Californian, if that's what you mean. Her family is originally from Peru, and her husband is from Texas, though I don't know where exactly. She communicates in a very direct style. I like that about her. I always know where we stand. She is totally honest, and she would never backstab anyone."

"But shoot them in the head?"

Robert chuckled. "If Dr. Díaz were to kill anyone, then it would probably be Dr. Oliver Robinson. The two don't get along."

"I noticed that."

"No, seriously: Dr. Díaz is not a killer. She might yell at you, but I don't think she would physically hurt anyone."

"You never know. I've learned over the years to not exclude anyone just based on their appearance. But there is a detail that I wanted to share with you: right before she was shot, Nia activated Siri, the online assistant on her iPhone, and said '*green eyes.*' We are wondering if this was a hint to identify the killer."

Robert looked at him. "Wow, that could help a lot. Green eyes are very rare. Less than 10% of the US population have it."

Terrel nodded. "It could be a first lead. Would your security team be able to produce a list of people on campus with green eyes?"

"That would be very easy," Robert responded. "Every new employee comes to see me or our chief of staff in this building. They all need to go through the iris scanner at the entrance. I will call our security team and get you a list right away."

"Thanks," Terrel said. "It could be helpful."

"You know that Dr. Annya Segond has green eyes?" the Dean said.

Terrel thought about it. Of course, Dr. Hill was right: Annya had light green eyes. But she was part of the law enforcement team. "Annya is one of us," Terrel said. "She worked for the CIA."

"Didn't the FBI chase her last year?" Dr. Hill remembered. "Her husband was a Russian spy?"

"Yes, that's true. Ex-husband. She helped us find him."

Dr. Hill shrugged. "You will have better resources to check this. She just came to my mind."

Terrel nodded. "Duly noted. I will check out everyone with green eyes, including Annya, and I won't stop with these people. I will scrutinize everyone who could have benefitted from Nia's death. Do you have any idea who could've done this? Any idea about the motive?"

Dean Hill shook his head. "I'm sorry. Until today, I didn't even know Nia."

Terrel made a few more notes in his notebook, then closed it and put it in his pocket. "Okay, I will talk with people on campus. Somebody must know something. And I will find the brother who Mrs. Johnes mentioned." He got up from his seat.

Robert remained seated. "Well, since you are here, perhaps we can discuss something else?"

Terrel looked at him. "What is that?"

The Dean pointed at the seat. "Would you mind sitting down for another minute, please? I would like to discuss a totally different, more personal matter."

Terrel looked at him in surprise. He sat down again.

Dean Hill produced a handkerchief and wiped his brows. "Well, I'm not sure how to begin."

This was getting interesting. Terrel leaned forward. "How about with the beginning? You know I deal with secrets all the time. Whatever it is, it's safe with me."

"Well, you might remember my husband, Atharv. We have been happily married for five years now. And we are about to adopt a baby."

"Congratulations!"

Robert sighed. "This past weekend, I attended a conference in Monterey. I had a very nice hotel room on the ground floor with a little patio that faced the beach. After the conference, I sat there enjoying a glass of wine and watching the sunset."

Terrel looked at him, trying to anticipate the plot.

"Suddenly, an Adonis comes by, jogging past my room with a bare chest and golden hair flying in the wind."

"Adonis—the Greek god of beauty?"

"You know what I mean. It was a very handsome young man. So, anyways, after a few minutes, this guy comes back. He stops at my patio and starts a conversation with me. One thing led to another. I might have offered him a glass of wine. He sat down, and we had an interesting conversation."

"You had an affair?"

"Well, the thing is, I do not remember what happened. I never had an affair in my life, and I would certainly not start one now. I love my husband! I believe this guy might have spiked my drink. I only had two glasses of wine. But I passed out!"

"You passed out? What do you remember?"

"We were talking on the patio. I felt a little tipsy. He was making jokes, we laughed. A lot. I felt hot and wanted to reach for a napkin. I got up and the world started spinning around. Then the lights went out. I lost consciousness. The next thing I know, I woke up in my bed without my clothes on."

"You were naked? And now you feel guilty?"

"I was horrified! And I cannot remember a thing."

"My condolences."

"Well, it did not end there. This morning, I got an email on my personal email account with photos." Dr. Hill swallowed.

Terrel could not suppress a smile. "Sounds like you were set up. Did your sender blackmail you?"

Robert Hill cleared his throat. "He wants me to step down from my role as SUEC Dean by Friday this week, or Atharv will get a copy."

"Wow. That is in two days from now. What will you do?"

"I will comply. I already prepared my resignation letter. Atharv is the love of my live, and he is very jealous. I cannot lose him over this stupid incident."

"Could you sit down with him and explain everything? If he truly loves you, he will understand. You were played."

Robert Hill shook his head. "It is more complicated. We are in the final phase of an adoption. The birthmother will deliver our baby on Saturday. A baby girl. She was hesitant to match with a gay couple at first. She thought we might not be able to raise her girl with moral values. But we convinced her of our integrity. If a scandal breaks, I am afraid she will change her mind. And Atharv would never forgive that. It would ruin our marriage."

"But if you give in to the blackmailer, you will lose a very powerful position."

Robert Hill shrugged. "What should I do? I am a researcher by heart. I will remain professor at SUEC and focus on what I love most—my research. I got into this administrative role by accident. I hate politics."

"I wonder if this incident is related to Nia's death. I would like to look into this. Can you please forward this email to me?"

"You cannot see the photos. I'm too embarrassed."

"I'm not judging you, Robert. My only concern is our national security. I want to see from which IP address this was sent to you. And I need a headshot from Adonis. We should be able to get that from the photo that was sent to you."

"Can you please promise that Atharv will not hear anything about this? And that nothing will leak to the press?"

"I will do the best I can." Terrel got up from his seat. "And please wait with your resignation letter. Perhaps this can be resolved without you stepping down. You have the highest integrity and are the humblest person I know. That must be good for the university, and it makes my life much easier."

Robert Hill got up as well. "Thank you so much, Terrel. I cannot tell you how much I appreciate your help."

"No problem. That's what I do." Terrel shook Dean Hill's hand, then turned around and walked back down the barrel-vaulted hallway, which still contained a lingering scent of Mrs. Johnes's magnolia perfume.

- 10 -

LILI

A Gun Shot
Wednesday, May 25, 2033, 10 am.

Lili dropped her empty paper cup in a trashcan on the hallway of the research building as she walked over to Dr. Robinson's lab. The lab consisted of an open space with five rows of benches and desks where an armada of young scientists was busy pipetting, preparing petri dishes, examining specimens under microscopes, handling samples on fuming dry ice, and entering data into computers. Lili looked around. Did all these people work with human embryos? That was a bit chilling.

She walked towards the person next to her, a young Asian man who was investigating a specimen on a glass slide under a microscope. "Hi, I am looking for Dr. Ingrid Maulvi. Do you know where I can find her?"

The man looked up and pointed to a young woman with double Dutch braids and ripped blue jeans who was sitting at a white desk in the next row. "Our program manager? She's over there."

Ingrid was sitting at a large linoleum desk close to the white-framed window, typing something on a computer. While all other desks in the room were shared by two people, hers was extra spacious, with one oversized chair and the largest computer in the room.

As Lili approached, Ingrid looked up. Her long dark braids embraced an angelic face with perfectly symmetric features, flawless light brown complexion, striking light blue eyes and cherry-red lipstick. Lili became painfully aware of her own messed-up appearance. No time for a blow-dry this morning. She straightened a rebellious strand of hair in front of her right eye with her fingers.

"Can I help you?" Ingrid asked with a low, authoritative voice. Lili looked at her with fascination. Ingrid's red-painted lips seemed to move autonomously. The rest of the face was not moving at all. Botox?

Lili pointed to the ID on her shirt. "Hi Ingrid, I'm a radiologist here at SUEC. You might have seen me before. I have a research lab on the first floor in this building."

Ingrid kept her eyes on the screen. "Would you like to start a collaboration? Oliver and I have a sign-up sheet for that," the red-lined mouth said.

"No, I thought you could help me out with a question."

Ingrid turned around and looked her up and down. Apparently, the result was not favorable. She turned back to her computer. "I'm sorry, but I'm really busy at the moment. Oliver and I have an important deadline for a patent coming up." She continued typing.

Lili cleared her throat. "Well, I was asked to review medical imaging studies from a research project. All patients had an infection and a history of IVF. Do you know anything about that project?"

"No, never heard of it." Ingrid continued typing.

"We believe it was Nia Johnes's project."

Ingrid looked up. "Is that so? Are you a private detective?"

"No, I'm just trying to make sense of these images."

Ingrid's gaze became intense, almost piercing. "Who gave you images of research patients?"

It would probably not be wise to mention Cristina here. "A CIA agent," Lili said, thinking of Annya, who had sent her the first images.

"The CIA is investigating Nia's death?"

"I guess so."

Ingrid flipped her right braid to her back. "And the CIA sent you here?"

"No, I'm just trying to understand what is going on. It seems that Nia was researching patients who were conceived with IVF. Would somebody here be collaborating on such a project?"

Ingrid shrugged. "I don't know anything about that. As I said, Oliver and I have an important deadline coming up. If you would excuse me now?" She turned away on her swiveling chair.

Lili looked at Ingrid's back. That was quite rude. She was a professor here. Even a colleague would not treat her so disrespectfully. Why was a lab manager acting like that?

After two decades in academia, Lili had learned that rudeness did not signify an offense, but leaked guilt. What was Ingrid hiding? "Ingrid, did you have pneumonia in the past few months?" Lili asked.

Ingrid looked back at her with her piercing gaze. "Did *I* have pneumonia?" she said with a tense tone. "Why are you asking that?"

Lili smiled. "One of the imaging studies had a note: *Ingrid*. Of course, it could've been a different Ingrid. I was just wondering…"

Ingrid interrupted her. "It was not me. And if I were you, I would be very careful," she said sharply. "What you are describing is a breach of patient privacy. If you are not involved in this research study, you should not have access to any patient names. Faculty can get fired for breaching patient privacy."

The situation was clearly getting hostile. Lili raised her hands. "I didn't mean to upset you, Ingrid. I think we are all on edge due to Nia's death. Thank you for chatting with me."

Ingrid's red-lined mouth formed a slight upwards curve without engaging the rest of her perfectly smooth face. "No problem. Have a good day!"

The door flung open, and a middle-aged man in black jeans, a white shirt, and an expensive-looking dark grey blazer walked into the room. All heads in the lab turned towards him, like a synchronized choreography in a ballet performance. Ingrid got up from her chair. "Good morning, Oliver!" she said with a flirty tone.

The man waved his open palm like a celebrity. "Hello, Ingrid, good to see you!" he said, smiling at her with a row of perfectly white teeth. Then, looking across the room, he said, "Hello, team, great to see you all!"

The heads nodded in acknowledgment and returned to fume hoods, lab benches, and computers while the man walked with long strides towards an office at the back end of the laboratory.

Lili looked at him. He was very handsome, with a palpable aura of authority. This had to be Prof. Dr. Oliver Stuart Robinson, director of this lab and Vice Dean of Academic Affairs at SUEC.

As he walked, he continued to scan the room, and stopped at Lili. She flushed. Had he caught her staring?

"Hello, Dr. Pham, what brings you here?" he said with a friendly tone.

Lili was surprised. As far as she could remember, she had not met him so far. But she had recently submitted her promotion paperwork, and Dr. Robinson was known to have an elephant memory. Some people said that he knew every single faculty member. Apparently, he did.

"Hello, Dr. Robinson, it is great to meet you in person!" Lili said politely. "I'm very impressed by your large lab."

He flashed his gleaming teeth again. "I'm glad you like it. Did you come to speak with me?" he asked.

"Yes!" Lili improvised. Since the discussion with Ingrid had been fruitless, why not talk with her boss?

"You are lucky. I have a few minutes before my first meeting today. Come this way." Dr. Robinson continued his path to his office, and Lili followed him. He pointed to the left. "These people here work on preparing fertilization reports and generating new methods of retrieving eggs from our patients." Lili nodded. He pointed to the right. "These people take care of sperm preparation for egg insemination and selecting embryos for an embryo transfer to a mother's uterus."

They had made their way down the aisle, and Dr. Robinson pointed to the left again. "These people freeze and thaw eggs, sperm, and embryos as needed."

Lili saw several young researchers in white lab coats pipetting, examining specimens under microscopes, and preparing cell culture dishes. Some of them looked up and waved at them briefly. Dr. Robinson waved back.

"The fastest way through the lab is to walk with someone else," he said in a low voice. "Then, nobody will ask us to stop and look at their presumed Nobel prize-winning discovery. Most of the time, it's not that ground-breaking. These kids just haven't seen much yet. But I admire their enthusiasm. That's what makes SUEC great!"

"I understand," Lili said.

Dr. Robinson pointed to the right. "These people here work on pre-implantation diagnosis."

A group of young people stood in front of three large PCR (polymerase chain reaction) machines, vortexing test tubes, entering samples into the machine, and recording the readouts.

Lili took in the whole scene. "How do you decide which embryos to implant, which to freeze, and which to discard?" she asked.

"Well, there are many factors. We investigate the DNA of eggs and embryos to select or exclude specific genes. It is useful when there are known genetic diseases in the family that should not be carried forward to the next generation and the next baby."

"Are embryos destroyed in the process?" Lili asked.

Dr. Robinson sent her a probing gaze. Lili returned an innocent smile. "Well, we typically create more embryos than we implant. The extra embryos can be frozen until patients choose to use them or donate them to another couple. The superfluous embryos can also be disposed of or donated to scientific research. Here in the United States, about 1-24% embryos are abandoned."

They had reached Dr. Robinson's office, a large, bright square room at the back end of the lab with a large floor-to-ceiling window that provided a great view towards the adjacent park. Dr. Robinson walked through the glass door that led into the office and made a gesture towards the left, where three gold-colored leather seats were situated in a half circle. They sat down. The golden color was a bit tacky, but the seat felt soft and comfortable. Lili looked around. To her right was a large mahogany desk with piles of neatly arranged files on it. *Perhaps promotion files*, she thought. *Including mine.*

Behind the desk, so dense that they covered the entire wall, were Dr. Robinson's diplomas and certificates mounted in ornamental gold and silver frames. Lili read: M.D. and Ph.D. degree from Harvard, residency training in obstetrics and gynecology at Stanford, fellowship in reproductive endocrinology at Stanford, Hendrikson Deanial Professor and Chair of the Department of Obstetrics and Gynecology at SUEC. *Impressive.*

"So, did you want to discuss your promotion application?" Dr. Robinson asked. "You know the process is confidential. I cannot really tell you anything."

Lili shook her head. "No, not at all. I did not come to talk about my promotion. I am well-prepared. I've published more than 150 publications and gotten three new research grants. Two of my colleagues were promoted recently with much less research activity."

Dr. Robinson leaned back in his chair. "Well, we do not just count publications and grants. The process is much more complex. As you know, we request letters from colleagues inside and outside of the university."

Lili nodded. She knew the drill. Over the past months, a lengthy dossier had been assembled about her, in which reviewers had been asked to subjectively judge her. The administrator who invited the letter writers could choose friends or foes, depending on the desired outcome. It was like a Yelp review where one person could invite all critics. This person was Dr. Robinson.

"Actually, I am here because of Nia Johnes. You might have heard that she was shot last night. I was contacted because she apparently collected medical imaging studies of patients with a history of IVF. All of the imaging studies showed infections. I was wondering if you know anything about her research project."

"No, I don't know anything about it. Nia collected medical images? Can you show them to me?"

Lili swallowed. Ingrid had reminded her that she was not supposed to look at any research data if she was not involved in that research. "Well, I only heard about it secondhand. Apparently, Nia collected medical images from patients with a history of IVF."

Dr. Robinson shrugged. "Well, it sounds like nothing concrete is known here. Be careful. When a student dies under questionable circumstances, people start to gossip."

Lili thought about an angle that would be acceptable. "FBI agent Terrel Wright is investigating the case. He mentioned that he found medical images from IVF patients in Nia's apartment."

"Is that so? Well, if none of our team members here was involved, I would question the scientific validity of that research. It is easy to just pick and choose data to support some propaganda. Unfortunately, there are still many people with prejudices against fertility treatment out there—including our friends next door."

"You know that Cristina Walker-Díaz has reservations against IVF?"

He smiled. "Of course, I do. Cristina shares her beliefs openly, often in a rather emotional manner. I have been trying to convince her that a more professional approach will be better for her career."

"She is a devoted Christian."

"She can believe what she wants. But she cannot enforce it on others. Do *you* think that we should impose Christian dogma on everyone on campus? Or all of our patients, for that matter?"

Lili shook her head. "Of course not. I would hope that we could respect each other, no matter what we believe—or not."

"Perhaps try to share that sentiment with Cristina. It seems that she is your friend."

"Yes, she is. And I feel so sorry for her. She is devastated about the death of her student."

"I am sorry to hear that. The well-being of our junior faculty is very important to SUEC. I'll stop by her office later today and see if I can offer some comfort."

Lili nodded. "Thank you, that is very kind of you. Do you have any idea why Nia would study IVF patients?"

"I don't know *if* she did that. It would not be in line with the research focus of her supervisor's lab, and it would not reflect well on Cristina if Nia did not follow her directions. Perhaps this is some kind of misunderstanding."

Lili nodded. She was starting to wonder the same. Perhaps she had missed something.

Dr. Robinson smiled. "And, by the way, we call fertility treatment more broadly 'assisted reproductive technology,' or ART. I prefer that term over IVF. We are artists here and are proud to deliver healthy babies every day!"

Lili was still processing the information provided to her. Why had Ingrid been so rude? Why did Dr. Robinson not ask what was on the medical images? Why did he talk about semantics with an SUEC student in the morgue? Who cared what IVF was called?

"Do you think Nia's research had something to do with her death?" she asked.

"I don't know anything about her research!" Dr. Robinson said sharply. The expression on his face morphed from friendly to serious. "Nia was not a member of my lab—or yours. This unfortunate death is none of our business. Let the police take care of it."

Lili did not know how to respond. Dr. Robinson must've seen Nia on a regular basis if she worked next door. How could he be so cold? Did he not have questions of his own?

Dr. Robinson cleared his throat. "Lili, let me give you some advice: You are at a critical point in your career. The evaluation letters for your promotion are currently being assembled. This is not just any promotion; this is an evaluation for tenure at SUEC. If this promotion goes through, you will have a lifetime appointment at the most famous university in the world. If you get negative evaluations, your position will not be extended, and you will lose your job. Do not get into any trouble at this important point in your career."

Lili felt a shiver down her spine. "Of course," she said calmly.

"I am glad we understand each other." Dr. Robinson stood up.

"Let the police do the detective job. That's what they are paid to do."

A dull throbbing sound filled the air.

A gun shot!

Lili jumped up and ran to the window. The sound came from somewhere below the window. There was a small grove with several tall rainbow eucalyptus trees. Their multicolored trunks extended high into the sky, and their leafy hanging branches obscured the view. Lili saw the two legs of a person on the ground. They wore ripped jeans, but she could not see their face. She stepped closer to the window to get a better view.

Dr. Robinson grabbed her arm and tried to pull her back. "Lili, get back from the window. If the shooter sees you, they might try to eliminate you as a witness. What did we just talk about?"

"The window is tinted—nobody can see us behind it," Lili responded. "It happened right below us. There's somebody lying on the ground, and several people are running towards them. Dr. Robinson, you must see this! I believe it might be Ingrid!"

"That can't be. She was in the lab just a few minutes ago." Dr. Robinson looked through his office glass door to the lab. Ingrid's desk was empty. He carefully stepped towards the window, trying to keep his body behind the window frame while finding a good spot to see the ground through the tree leaves. "Indeed, it is Ingrid!" he exclaimed.

He turned around and rushed out of the room. Lili followed him closely. They ran through the lab. The students there looked up wearily. Some went to the window to see what was going on, and others followed their boss. Dr. Robinson hurried down the hallway, down the stairs, through the atrium, and around the building to the spot that they had seen from the window. Lili followed him closely, along with several other researchers.

A small crowd had assembled below the multi-colored eucalyptus trees. Ingrid was sitting on the ground, examining her right arm. The shoulder area of her jacket was soaked in blood.

Thank God she's alive! Several witnesses were taking photos with their cell phones. Lili couldn't help but think that these photos would go viral on social media.

Dr. Robinson kneeled beside her. "Ingrid, what happened?" he asked with a fearful tone. "Are you hurt?"

"I don't know," she responded softly. "I heard a shot, and

suddenly felt a sharp pain in my arm. I believe somebody shot at me."

Lili pushed herself through the crowd. "I am a physician! Let me have a look."

Ingrid looked at her with that same spark in her pretty blue eyes that Lili had noticed earlier. She couldn't quite interpret what it meant. It was definitely not fear—more like anger.

"Can you remove your jacket, please?" Lili asked. Ingrid did as she was asked. Lili and Dr. Robinson examined the arm carefully. The underlying blouse had a small horizontal defect, and the skin of the left upper arm was scratched, with blood around it. "It's just a superficial injury, " Lili concluded. "You're fine."

Dr. Robinson shook his head. "I don't think so. And, for legal purposes, we have to document the extent of your injury. Ingrid, I will call the emergency room at SUEC hospital. They must examine you."

"Thank you, Oliver," Ingrid responded with an upwards gaze.

They heard heavy boot steps and breathing sounds approaching. Lili looked up and saw FBI Agent Terrel Wright running towards them. He stopped in front of them, panting. "What happened here?" he asked, catching his breath.

"I was shot!" Ingrid cried.

"Shot by whom?" Terrel asked. He looked around. A small group of people had assembled around Ingrid, but there was no runner anywhere. Nobody who looked suspicious.

"I don't know," Ingrid said. "I believe the shooter was hiding behind the trees." She pointed to the right, at the eucalyptus trees in the park, which were surrounded by rhododendron bushes.

Terrel stepped towards the park area. There was nobody. He turned to the small group of people around Ingrid. "Nobody leaves," he said with an authoritative voice. "I would like to talk with each and every one of you. Think carefully whether you saw anything or anyone suspicious. If you have any personal identification with you, please have it ready."

Lili looked around and counted. There were about fifteen people in addition to Ingrid, herself, and Dr. Robinson. Three security guards had arrived at the scene as well. Terrel asked one of them to record the names and contact information of all the spectators. He asked the other two to search the premises for suspicious people and a gun. Then he spoke with Ingrid and Dr. Robinson.

The security guard asked Lili and several others to step back and wait for their turn to speak with the FBI agent. She sat down on a park bench. It was eerily calm here. She looked over her shoulder. Hopefully, the shooter was not hiding in the rhododendron bushes.

After a while, Terrel, Ingrid, and Dr. Robinson parted. Another security guard appeared with a small electric car, Ingrid got in, and they drove away. Dr. Robinson disappeared through the entrance of the research building, and Terrel walked towards Lili. "Hi, Lili, what were *you* doing here?" he greeted her.

"I have a research day today and my lab is in this building."

"Did you see anything unusual? Anything that could help us find the shooter?"

"I was meeting with Dr. Robinson when we heard the gunshot. His office is right above this area here." Lili pointed upwards. Dr. Robinson's office was indeed right above them. And it was indeed not possible to see through the tinted glass facade. "I was right there." She pointed at the window. "But I'm afraid I did not see anything. It all happened too fast."

"I understand," Terrel said. "What did you see?"

"I heard a gunshot. It seemed to come from the park. I looked out of the window and saw Ingrid lying on the ground. I did not see anybody else. The trees might have covered the shooter. Several people came running from the street. I ran down to her as well. That's all."

He sat down beside her. "How do you know Ingrid?" he asked.

Lili felt herself blushing. Cristina had specifically asked her not to say anything about the imaging studies, and she did not want to get in trouble for having reviewed some. "Well, Ingrid works in the same research building as I. I talked with her earlier this morning to see if she knows anything about Nia's death."

Terrel smiled. "So, you played detective? Did you find anything interesting?"

Lili shook her head. "Not really. Apparently, Nia studied infections of patients who had a history of in vitro fertilization. I don't think that was so groundbreaking that somebody would shoot her."

"And Ingrid."

"Yeah, I cannot quite put it together. What do the two women have in common? Or did they work together on this ominous research project? But Ingrid denied that she knew anything about it."

Terrel looked at her. "You work here. Do you have any suspicion who the shooter might be?"

Lili shook her head again. "No, I am afraid, I have no clue.

"Did you notice anyone on campus or in the research building today, or over the past few days, who did not belong here?"

Lili thought about it. "I saw some tourists on guided tours on the visitor promenade. You might remember, we have two different promenades here that lead from the entrance gate to the main university building on the top of the hill. Tourists go on guided tours up and down the visitor's promenade, which does not connect to the research buildings. They never get here. Visiting scientists or delivery personnel are only allowed to enter the research buildings with an SUEC staff member. So, it would be quite difficult for strangers to come here without being noticed."

Terrel made some notes in his notebook. "I see. I will check with the front gate staff who checked in today and in the last two to three days. Who did you see in the research building this morning?"

Lili thought for a moment. "I saw Cristina Walker-Díaz, Jacub Bezdomny, Ingrid Maulvi, and Oliver Stuart Robinson. I saw my own team members in the lab. I also saw a few other students and postdoctoral fellows whose names I don't know."

"Are you aware of any hot new research in this building that would be worth killing for?"

Lili shrugged. "Well, we have several Nobel prize winners in this building, but their research was not targeted here. Cristina is still junior faculty, but she received multiple awards already for her work on personalized drug therapies. She complained that Nia was not making much progress with her research in her lab. And if anyone would have been interested in Cristina's research, wouldn't they have attacked her? I really have no clue what this is about."

"Understood." Terrel took a few more notes, then looked up at her. "Is there anything else that comes to mind regarding this case?"

"Well, Cristina mentioned that Nia had a list of IVF patients, which somehow disappeared. This could be unrelated, or perhaps Nia discovered some sensitive information. Still, I cannot imagine that anyone would kill her over a research project. Perhaps her death is completed unrelated."

Terrel nodded. "Our team will look at every angle. Thanks for helping me out here, Lili. It's great that you work here. I remember you have a very keen eye. Please go back to the lab and call me if you notice anything out of the ordinary. You've still got my phone number?"

"Yes, I do!"

"Okay, you are dismissed." He smiled.

"Thanks!" Lili smiled as well.

In her next life, she would become an FBI agent.

- 11 -

ANNYA

The Exam
Wednesday, May 25, 2033, 1 p.m.

Annya ran to the entrance of the emergency room. Two nurses followed her closely. She had received a text message from FBI agent Terrel Wright that another gunshot victim was on the way to the hospital. The security guard in front of the ER had cleared the entrance area to make space for an arriving ambulance.

When Annya stepped on the square in front of the hospital, she saw a small self-driving electric car with a large SUEC sign approaching. It looked more like a golf cart than an ambulance. A young woman and a young man were sitting on the back seat, engaged in a lively discussion. The woman was leaning back against the cushioned backseat, her left arm resting on the window frame. She looked at the man and laughed. There was no sign of distress on her face or her companion's. Annya's experienced eyes told her in a split second that these people did not need urgent medical attention. The cart stopped in front of her.

"Did you want to check in to the emergency room?" she asked the driver.

The young man looked at her: "Yes, we need urgent help! Dr. Maulvi here was shot on the SUEC campus."

Annya looked at the young woman in front of her. She was adjusting her sunglasses and looking back at Annya with a relaxed smile. There were no signs of distress on her face, let alone any sign of a gunshot wound. Her cheeks were rosy, her lips outlined with fresh dark red lipstick. There were a few eucalyptus leaves in her silky black braids. *Very decorative.* "What is the medical problem?" Annya asked calmly.

The woman pointed at her left upper arm. "I was shot this morning. Fortunately, the shooter almost missed."

"Dr. Maulvi works for Dr. Stuart Robinson," her companion explained. "You know, the Vice Dean. He asked that she be examined here. The results should be documented for an official report."

Annya looked at the man. He wore silver SUEC overalls, so probably a staff person. "And you are?" she asked.

"I am an SUEC security guard. Dr. Robinson asked me to make sure that Dr. Maulvi arrived here safely. Fortunately, we did not encounter any additional shooting incidents on our way here."

"I understand," Annya responded, thinking, *An FBI examiner could have taken care of this.* This woman surely needed an interview and an exam for documentation, but she did not need urgent care.

And Annya, of all people, should know. She remembered how her estranged husband had shot her in a rant of jealousy. She had fought for her life in the ICU. She hadn't known at the time that he was a Russian spy. That revelation had brought her to the CIA.

But that was a long time ago. And her ex-husband was dead now.

Annya looked at the young woman again. "Come this way," she said. Ingrid Maulvi followed her to the exam room.

Annya noted that there was a small hole in Ingrid's jacket. She opened a drawer and took out a silver SUEC T-shirt. "Here, you can wear this," she said. "I will need your jacket and T-shirt for forensic examinations. Where were you when you were hit?"

"I was standing in the park beside the SUEC research building," Ingrid responded. She had taken off her sunglasses and looked at Annya with piercing ice-blue eyes.

Annya sat down at her desk and took notes in Ingrid's file on the computer. Then, she asked Ingrid to sit down on the stretcher and examined her arm carefully, taking photos of the small wound and wiping it with cotton swabs. It was more of a scratch than anything. Annya sealed the swabs in plastic tubes and handed them over to a nurse. "Please send these to the forensic lab for analysis of gunshot residues with flameless atomic absorption spectrometry and scanning electron microscopic-energy dispersive x-ray spectrometry."

The nurse nodded and left the room.

"I hope you'll find something," Ingrid said. "I have to say that I cleaned the wound with an alcohol wipe."

"Is that so? Did you not know that that could eliminate evidence? You work in a medical research lab, right?"

"I'm sorry. That's why I'm telling you now. I was in shock and wanted to clean up the blood and prevent an infection."

"I see."

The wipes would be useless. Annya made another note in the medical file and placed a Band-Aid over the wound. "The wound looks clean. It will heal in no time."

"Thank you for looking at it. I appreciate your help. This was quite a shock, you know. When I heard the gunshot and felt the pain, I thought I was going to die. At first, I didn't know if it was my chest or my arm. Then, I noticed that my arm was bleeding."

"Through the jacket?"

"Yeah, something was running down my arm. I put my hand on it under the jacket, and when I looked at it, I saw that it was blood. You see some blood stains on the jacket as well now, but it probably took some time to soak through."

"I see. And you know it was a bullet because you heard a gunshot."

"Yeah. What else could it be?"

"You tell me. I am just trying to understand what happened. Are you sure that a bullet struck you?"

"Well, I mean, I am not absolutely sure. I've never been shot at before. I fell backwards, and it is also possible that my arm hit a tree branch or a sharp object on the ground."

The women's hair braids were meticulous. It was hard to believe that this head had struck anything. Annya made another note in the file. "And you have no clue whatsoever who could have done this? You are a very smart woman; you must have some suspicion."

"Well, I don't want to raise any false accusations."

"Ingrid, I'm an emergency physician. I am concerned about your safety. You might have escaped this time, but who knows what happens next time? Nia was killed last night. There's clearly a shooter out there who has no scruples."

"I don't have any enemies."

"The most common reasons for deadly shooting incidents are robbery, jealousy, and vengeance. Does any of that ring a bell?"

Ingrid flipped back her shimmering hair braids. "Well, I have a very good relationship with Oliver—I mean, Dr. Robinson. You know, I practically run his lab, and we meet regularly to discuss the progress of our research. Jacub, the research building manager, does not seem to like that. He often looks at me with this creepy gaze. You know, the kind of gaze that scans your body up and down. I'm pretty sure he has some sort of crush on me. And he often appears out of nowhere when I'm meeting with Oliver. I've wondered if he's jealous."

"Did Jacub ever threaten you in any way?"

"I don't think he's dangerous, if that's what you mean. He's just weird. Oliver and I often have to work late at night because the fertilization procedures in the lab have to follow precise schedules. Jacub is often in the building until late at night. As if he were waiting for me."

"That does sound unsettling."

"Yeah, now that you bring that up, I noticed that he's followed Cristina Walker-Díaz as well. He is stalking women. He had been homeless for some time. Perhaps he has mental health issues. You never know what is going on in people's heads."

"Terrel Wright will contact me later today to receive my report about your exam. I can mention your concern to him. Or you can tell him yourself."

"I would appreciate if you would let him know. I do not want to undergo another interrogation today. I am exhausted. But it might be a good idea if the FBI agent could check Jacub out."

"I understand. I will let Agent Wright know."

"If it's okay, I'll take the rest of the day off. I do not want to return to the university campus today. I do not feel safe there."

Annya nodded. "I understand. From a medical point of view, you can go home now."

Ingrid played with her braids. "I have one last question."

"What is that?"

"When you look at my file, you will see that I had a tuberculosis infection some time ago. I recovered, but, as you know, tuberculosis has a high stigma around here. When I was sick, people did not want to come near me. And even after I had been successfully treated, they were afraid I could infect them. I would appreciate if you could keep this information private. Please do not share it with anyone."

"I will do the best I can. I have to release information if it is crucial for an investigation that involves our national security. I don't think this is the case here, but I want you to know that there can be exceptions to patient privacy rules."

Ingrid got up from her stretcher. "I understand. Please just keep my medical information private unless such an exception would come up."

"Of course." Annya closed the electronic medical record system.

Annya and Ingrid left the exam room together. Annya showed Ingrid the way from the ER suite to the electrical vertical take-off and landing station in front of the hospital. Ingrid walked over to the passenger waiting area and Annya walked back to her office. Through the window, she could see Ingrid entering the eVTOL aircraft, which took off and flew towards the city.

Annya dialed Terrel's number. He picked up right away. "Hello?"

"Hi, Terrel, I just saw your second victim, or presumed victim, Ingrid Maulvi."

"What do you mean?"

"Well, I'm pretty sure that the wound I have been looking at was not created by a gunshot. I took some photos, and I also collected the jacket and shirt. The holes in her clothes don't look like gunshot injuries either. Your forensic team can confirm that."

"I'm not sure I can follow. Are you saying she was not shot at?"

"I don't know that. Perhaps the shooter missed, and she fell and just scratched her arm or something. But it is odd that the wound is so clean. It didn't look like a cut from a tree branch or rose bush in the park; it looked more like a knife cut."

"Self-inflicted injury?"

"I wondered about that."

"Hm, that would also explain why nobody saw the shooter. This incident happened in the middle of the day and a lot of people were around. I interviewed about twenty witnesses. But nobody saw anyone walking or running away from the crime scene."

"But why would she fake a shooting incident?"

"Perhaps to distract us? I certainly didn't find the time to have a closer look at this lab of Dr. Robinson's. Nia investigated patients who have been conceived by IVF. There must be some connection to that lab."

"And someone in that lab is busy hiding it."

"Exactly."

"Oh, speaking of distractions: Ingrid mentioned that she thinks that the building manager might have targeted her.”

“Jacub? My impression so far is that he is nosy, but I don’t think he’s dangerous.”

“Yeah, it might be a red herring. But you never know. If you’re there right now, you could have a closer look at him.”

“I wanted to do that anyways. Apparently, he delivered a toothpaste to Nia last night. I just got a call from the forensic team saying that it contained high quantities of ketamine.”

“A sedative drug? That could explain witness reports that Nia’s car was zigzagging and driving much below the speed limit. Some witnesses reported that they saw Nia driving with her face very close to the windshield.”

“So, she was likely drugged. But if Jacub spiked the toothpaste, he wouldn’t have told me about it himself.”

“Perhaps someone wanted to frame him.”

“We’ll see. I still have to interview two more witnesses about the shooting incident here. Then I’ll head over to him.”

“I’m glad we talked!”

“Always a pleasure working with you, Annya! And your friend Lili. Together, we will find the shooter in no time.”

Annya hesitated for a moment. “Last time, you worked with a colleague, Agent Weber?”

“Yes, I did.”

“Do you still work with him?”

“Yes. He is my boss. If this turns out to be a case of national security, he might get involved.”

“That’s good to know.”

“Why do you ask for Angus?” Terrel asked. “Am I not enough?”

Annya sighed. “Terrel, come on. I only know you as partners. If Angus were the only one to investigate, I would have asked for you.”

“Of course.”

- 12 -

HEINZ

The Connection
Wednesday, May 25, 2033, 1 p.m.

Heinz was sitting at the desk in his home office when he received Ingrid's text message. *Nia was shot dead last night.*

He couldn't believe his eyes. He called Ingrid on her cell phone, but she didn't respond.

He googled "woman shot dead in San Francisco" and hit the "Last 24 Hours" tab. A brief article in the *San Francisco Chronicle* popped up, with Nia's photo in it. It was her!

He read the headline: *SUEC researcher shot on the 101 highway.* Heinz was overwhelmed. He had just found his sister. And now he lost her? His eyes welled with tears, and he groaned in pain. Schnitzel got up from his favorite daytime spot below the window, where the sun sent warm rays into the room. He tapped over to Heinz and placed his head in his lap. Heinz stroke the dog's head gently.

He remembered Nia's smile. How she threw back her head and laughed when he said something funny. How excited Schnitzel was every time he saw her. How she ruffled Schnitzel's head. How she had been standing on their doorstep last night, not quite herself. *What on earth happened?*

Heinz read the rest of the article. Not much more information there, really. Nia was shot last night, and the shooter got away. A person in a black motorcycle suit. They did not even know if it was a man or a woman. The police were investigating the case. There was a phone number that people could call to provide information that could help finding the shooter. Heinz wrote down the number. Perhaps he would call them later. This had to have something to do with the laptop that Nia brought him yesterday.

Heinz fetched the laptop and opened it again. Nia had been really nervous about it last night. But there was not much on it—some data from a research project. Who would care about that? Heinz randomly opened a file on the screen. It was just another CT scan. He read the note that was attached to it: Patient 12. Mucormycosis after COVID-19.

Mucormycosis? What was that? Heinz googled the term. He learned that mucormycosis were fungi commonly found in decaying organic substances. The spores of the fungi could be inhaled and caused infections of the sinus, the cavities around the nasal pathways, and the lungs. Most of the time, a patient's own immune system could fight the infection off, but in case of a compromised immune system, mucormycosis could cause major destructions of the infected organs.

Heinz looked at the CT scan. Indeed, there was a large hole in the lung. Even he could see that. He continued reading the notes for this case: *This image shows a characteristic bird's nest sign, a lesion with a very thick rim with a lucent center, which is fairly suggestive of the diagnosis of mucormycosis. This infection resolved completely.*

What was this all about? Heinz could not wrap his head around it. Why had Nia been so nervous about these cases? Why had she brought him the laptop in the middle of the night? Apparently, she did not trust her colleagues in her lab. Otherwise, she had given the laptop to one of them. But instead, she had asked Heinz to delete the tracking function and backup system of the computer so that nobody would find it. What was so hot about these cases that somebody would kill her for it? Nia, the most kind and gentle person he knew.

Heinz shook his head. This made no sense at all.

He opened the next file. Patient 13. Mucormycosis after COVID-19. Heinz opened the attached note: *CT images of the lung show a focal lesion in the right upper lung, with a thick rim and lucent center, consistent with mucormycosis. The lesion resolved on follow up imaging scans.*

Heinz opened another file. This was a patient list. Patient numbers, age, gender, different disease diagnoses, clinical outcomes. He scrolled through it. *What's so interesting about it?*

The doorbell rang. Heinz closed the laptop and went down the stairs with Schnitzel in tow. It was Ingrid. She did not look sad. But then, she was just extremely composed in all situations. It was hard to see any emotion on her face at any time.

"Hello, Heinz," she said calmly, flipping her right braid back.

"Hello." Heinz looked at her. It was mind-boggling that this delicate, stunning woman was related to him. They were complete antitheses of each other: He oversized, shy, introverted, and she slim, confident, commanding. The only things they had in common were their light blue eyes.

Schnitzel appeared beside Heinz. He looked at Ingrid, growled, and showed his teeth. Ingrid stepped back. Schnitzel moved towards her and growled more loudly. "Schnitzel, stop it!" Heinz grabbed him by his collar, pulled him into the adjacent kitchen, and closed the door.

"Sorry," he said to Ingrid with a mischievous smile. "I don't know why he's doing that."

Ingrid looked at him with a serious expression. "Don't worry about the dog. Perhaps I have some scent from the lab on me that he does not like. Did you get my message about Nia?"

Heinz nodded. "I did. I couldn't believe it at first. Nia is dead!" He swallowed.

"I'm so sorry, Heinz. I know she meant a lot to you."

"Did you know she was in trouble?"

"I had no idea. But that is really no street conversation." Ingrid looked back as a homeless man walked by with his cart. She waved two paper bags. "I brought sandwiches. Did you have lunch yet?"

"No, I forgot to eat with all this. I'm not sure I'm hungry. Would you like to come in?"

Ingrid nodded. "This is a terrible situation, but we have to eat. We don't want to die of starvation." She flung her arm around Heinz's shoulders, making him melt. They walked inside and over to the living room in the rear end of the house. Ingrid sat down on the large leather couch and placed the paper bags on the ottoman in front of her. Heinz opened the white framed French doors. A cool summer breeze came in, carrying the scent of jasmine from the backyard.

Schnitzel barked in the kitchen and scratched at the door. Heinz went back, slowly opening the door. "Sit!" he demanded with a serious tone. Schnitzel sat immediately, staring at him intently, his tail wagging.

Heinz fetched two plates and two LaCroix sodas, and then looked at Schnitzel again. "Stay!" He walked back to the living room, the dog following closely. When the dog saw Ingrid, he growled again. Heinz sat on one of two matching leather seats opposite the couch. He pointed at a plush pet bed beside his seat. "Schnitzel, stay here."

Schnitzel hesitated at first, looking at Ingrid, the paper bags, and Heinz. But then he sat obediently on the pet bed, staring intently at Ingrid. Heinz pointed at the hallway with his index finger. "If you misbehave, I'll put you back into the kitchen!"

The dog tilted his head, looking at him. Then, he settled down, placing his large head on Heinz's feet, still following Ingrid's every move with his eyes. Ingrid smiled. "Perhaps he's jealous!"

"Maybe." Heinz looked at his dog. Schnitzel had behaved completely differently with Nia. "Whatever it is, he will have to learn to accept you. You are part of our family now."

Heinz handed Ingrid a plate and soda. She took the soda. He reached for a sandwich. Grilled ham, cheese, and tomatoes with lots of Dijon mustard, his favorite. Heinz started eating. The sandwich did not taste good today. His grieving mind could not be lulled so easily. He sighed. *Everything* was bitter today.

Ingrid opened the soda can with a pop. She took a sip and looked around. Heinz followed her gaze to the bookcases to their right. "Real books?" she asked.

"Real books!" he confirmed with a smirk. "A heritage from my parents."

"They were from Canada?"

"Yes, my father was from Ottawa, and my mother was from Germany. They met at McGill University and decided to stay in Montreal. I grew up there. But they both died a few years ago, during the COVID-19 pandemic."

"I'm very sorry. I didn't know that."

"Yeah, it was a very difficult time. I do not have any other siblings and was very lonely. I got very depressed. My primary care physician suggested that I get a dog. So, I went to an animal shelter and found Schnitzel there. He was very young, and as depressed as I was. His previous owner had abandoned him. We became instant friends. From there, everything got better." Heinz ruffled Schnitzel's head. Schnitzel closed his eyes and leaned into him.

"How did you end up here in San Francisco?" Ingrid asked.

"A few months after I adopted Schnitzel, my aunt, who lived in this house, died as well, at the age of 101 years. My parents and I had visited her every summer, and I loved it here. To my surprise, she put me on her deed. So, we moved here."

Heinz looked at Ingrid. "How about you? You mentioned that you grew up in the Bay Area?"

Ingrid took a sip from her soda. "Yes, I did. My grandparents immigrated from India to Berkeley when my mother was only five years old. She met my father here. His great-grandparents immigrated from Denmark to Solvang. You know, that small village close to Santa Barbara."

"I visited it once. A beautiful little town. I loved the windmills and the bakeries there!"

Ingrid nodded. "Yeah, you could smell the fresh bread from two blocks away. We visited our grandparents often when I was a kid. Those were good times."

Heinz had almost finished his sandwich. He handed a piece of ham to Schnitzel, who gratefully accepted. "You mentioned that you lost a parent as well?"

"Yeah, my dad died of COVID when I was fifteen years old. Our entire family had COVID. My mother and I recovered, although we both suffered from long term consequences. My mother got brain fog and struggled to take care of me as a single mom. She worked part-time, and we had a very hard time making ends meet. I got an injury of my olfactory nerve and facial nerve. I lost my ability to smell and taste. And I can barely move the muscles of my forehead anymore."

"I am sorry. I always thought you were very composed. I did not think that you had a disability."

"Yeah, it affects every aspect of my life. People judge me because I do not notice the fragrance of flowers, food, or people around me. I cannot smell or taste if food has gone bad. It is quite devastating."

Heinz looked at his dog. "Perhaps this is one reason why Schnitzel behaves so strangely around you."

"Perhaps," Ingrid responded. "Or perhaps German Shepherds are just very protective of their owners. I actually like that about your dog. He watches out for you."

Heinz ruffled Schnitzel's head again. "We watch out for each other," he said softly. The dog looked up at him, his wet nuzzle moving closer. Perhaps there was an opportunity here to get another bite.

Heinz turned back towards Ingrid. "Why are you not at work today?" he asked. "Did you take time off after you heard about Nia?"

Ingrid took a tiny bite from her sandwich. "Someone shot at me in the park behind the research building," she said, chewing.

"What?" Heinz stared at her. "You were shot at as well? And you only mention this now?" He looked at Ingrid's blank face.

"Yeah, it was quite a shock in the moment. But I'm fine, really. The shooter missed me. The bullet hardly scratched my arm. Oliver—my supervisor—sent me to the emergency room. The ER physician there examined me, put a bandage on the wound, and sent me home."

Heinz wiped sweat beads from his forehead. "This is horrible. Who shot at you?" he asked. "Do you think it was the same person who shot Nia?"

"I don't know. The emergency physician asked the same thing."

"Do you know anyone who might want to harm you?"

Ingrid shook her head. "I have no enemies. I mean, some people don't like me, but I don't know anyone who would want to *kill* me. I can only imagine that this was an accident. Presumably, that person wanted to shoot somebody else, and I was just in the way."

Heinz moved to the edge of his seat. "This is terrible, Ingrid! I cannot lose another dibling. I cannot!"

Ingrid nodded. "Yeah, I do feel a little uncomfortable going home right now. I wondered if I could stay here with you today? Just one night? Or maybe two? Hopefully, the shooter will be caught soon by the police. I heard even the FBI is on the case."

Heinz swallowed. He looked at the gorgeous woman in front of him. These were awful circumstances, but he felt really lucky right now. "Of course," he said lightly. "You can have the guest room upstairs and can stay if you like.

"Thank you so much, Heinzi!" Ingrid said. "I feel so much safer here with you. And if anyone dared to come here, I'm sure Schnitzel would chase them away."

Schnitzel's head went towards her when he heard his name. He looked at her and growled again. "I'm sure we will become friends, Schnitzel!" she said with a soothing voice. "Can I offer you my sandwich?" She got up from the couch and walked over to the dog.

Schnitzel looked at her and the sandwich—the sandwich in her hand, the sandwich on the move, the sandwich on the floor in front of him. He sniffed at it. It smelled good. He decided to eat it.

Heinz chuckled. "I believe you convinced him."

- 13 -

LILI

The Revelation
Wednesday, May 25, 2033, 2 p.m.

After her discussion with Terrel Wright, Lili went back into the SUEC research building. When she entered the foyer, she saw Oliver Stuart Robinson coming from the bathrooms on the left and Cristina Walker-Díaz walking down the spiral staircase. Lili stopped and held her breath. The trajectories of the two adversaries would inevitably cross.

Dr. Robinson noticed her first. "Hello, Cristina! It is nice to see you!" he said with a cheery tone.

Cristina looked at him briefly. "Pardon, I cannot say the same." She walked past him.

"I am sorry for the death of your student," he said to her back. "I hope you can find comfort in your belief that this was God's plan."

Cristina turned around. "*You* are sorry?" she said. "I am not sure about that. Nia studied infections in patients with IVF. Isn't it convenient for you that this project ended? And it is deeply offensive to suggest that this was God's plan for a young student."

"You are being hurtful, Cristina."

She pointed her index finger at him. "*You* are being hurtful, Oliver. And you do not even notice it! You are unable to empathize with anyone but yourself."

He put his hands in his pockets, looking at her with a mischievous smile. "Are you suggesting that I am insensitive, Cristina?"

"You are self-centered, Oliver. I'm sorry if that is news to you. I really thought you already knew."

"How selfish or selfless I am might be a matter of opinion."

"Oh, you don't like my opinion? You should hear the ones I keep to myself."

He raised his hands. "Cristina, I know that this is a very difficult situation for you right now, but you are SUEC faculty. You cannot act so weird in public."

She scoffed. "I'm not weird. I am just outside your exceptionally narrow point of view."

"You are insulting me, Cristina. But this is not about me. You are grieving the loss of your student."

Cristina raised her index finger again. "This is *very much* about *you*, Oliver! If Nia had not studied *your* patients, then she would still be alive!"

"What are you talking about?" Oliver responded calmly. "Cristina, you are creating stories in your mind that have nothing to do with reality. I am concerned that you are not well."

"The only thing that is wrong with me is that I'm talking with you right now," she responded in a high-pitched voice. "Leave me alone!" She turned around and walked out of the building.

Lili's jaw had dropped. She had never heard anyone talking so boldly to Dr. Robinson. He was the most powerful man on campus. Of course, Dr. Robert Hill was the SUEC Dean, but as such, Dr. Hill's responsibilities focused on the world outside of the SUEC campus: public relations, industry negotiations, donor interactions, and the like. Meanwhile, Dr. Robinson was the undisputed king of the SUEC community. Nobody—faculty, staff, or student—got anywhere without his blessing and approval. Cristina was only an assistant professor. She had many career advancements in front of her, all of which had to be approved by Dr. Robinson, so her outburst here was close to academic suicide.

Lili saw Jacub coming down the stairs. *Did he see this interaction as well?*

Jacub reached the base of the stairs, where Dr. Robinson was still standing. Jacub politely greeted him. The Vice Dean looked at him in perfect composure. "Hello, Jacub, would you fetch me an Arnold Palmer?" he said calmly.

Jacub nodded. "Certainly, Dr. Robinson. I will bring it to your office."

"Thank you!" The Vice Dean turned around, walked swiftly up the stairs, and disappeared on the second-floor hallway.

Two students in the corner of the foyer had stepped into the shadows of the adjacent research tract. They now quietly rushed through the entrance hall.

Lili walked over to Jacub. "Did you see that?" she asked in a low voice.

"Perhaps I did," he whispered. "Or perhaps I didn't. I don't want to get in trouble over other people's issues. Especially if they have the power to fire me with a snap of their fingers."

"Of course." Lili nodded. "I just don't understand why Cristina would act like that."

Jacub smirked. "Cristina is emotional. She is trying to hold everything in, but when the right trigger comes along, she just explodes, and all of her emotions come out at once."

"And that trigger is Dr. Robinson? I understand that she does not like his work on IVF. But that alone does not explain what we just saw here."

Jacub shrugged. "Well, they had an affair," he said in a low voice.

"Cristina and Oliver Robinson?" Lili burst out in disbelief.

Jacub put his index finger on his lips. "*Pst.* Remember, we are in the lobby here," he whispered.

Lili looked around. "There is nobody here right now," she whispered back. "This is unbelievable, and completely inappropriate! How do *you* know about it?"

Jacub shrugged. "Well, I see a lot of things here. Most people treat me like air."

"And what happened exactly?"

"This was about two years ago, when Cristina had just started working here. I thought she was the most stunning woman at SUEC, and apparently, Dr. Robinson thought so as well. I assume Cristina did not know about his IVF research at the time. I saw them kissing here in the foyer late at night. A few weeks later, they behaved like cats and dogs. I assumed that was the end of it."

Lili nodded. "They did sound like an estranged couple, indeed."

Jacub shrugged again. "As I said: Not my business, but if I must take sides, I am on team Cristina!"

"I really hope it does not come to us taking sides. But I wonder about what she said. If somebody is angry, people often do not hear their message. I always found this perplexing—if somebody is very emotional when they say something, it might be really important."

"I know what you mean," Jacub said. "Cristina said that Nia's research on Dr. Robinson's patients killed her."

"Exactly! Do you know why she would say that?"

Jacub scratched his head. "Again, I don't want to get sucked into some drama—or risk my life."

Lili looked at him. "But you noticed something else?"

"Yeah. About two weeks ago, Nia spent the entire night on the PCR machine. Making sure the PCR machine runs without any technical issues is one of my responsibilities—during the daytime of course. When she went for a bathroom break, I slipped into the lab and made a few copies of her results, just in case somebody complained the next day that there was a technical issue. Apparently, she did some DNA analyses of herself, Ingrid Maulvi, Dr. Robinson, and a few others whose names I did not recognize. I did not understand what the results showed. But I kept the copy, just in case. In the following days, I did not get any complaint about the PCR machine, and so, I forgot about the whole business."

"Do you still have these copies?"

"I guess so. I took photos with my iPhone. And I did wonder if I should hand them over to the FBI agent who was here this morning, but again, I do not want to get sucked into any issues."

Lili pointed to the iPhone in Jacub's front pocket. "If you have the photos on your phone now, could you just Airdrop them to me? I won't tell anyone where I got them."

Jacub looked at her for a moment. Then, he took his phone and typed something.

A few seconds later, Lili's phone beeped to indicate an incoming message. She accepted it and looked through the files. "I don't know what this is either, but I will find out," she said.

Jacub put his phone back into his pocket. "Thanks, Lili! I hope it helps find the shooter. But please remember to keep me out of it."

"Of course! Thanks for being so vigilant, Jacub. If we all keep our eyes open, we will find that bastard and bring him to justice!"

Lili turned around and stepped through the sliding glass doors into the open forecourt of the building. The California sun sat high in the spotless blue sky and the heat of the midday hit her like a dragon's breath. The path in front of the research building was desolate. A group of students had settled under the shades of the eucalytus trees to her right. A light breeze carried the sweet smell of eucalyptus and jasmin to her. Lili looked around. Cristina would know what these PCR results meant. But where had she gone?

Lili turned towards the park, where Terrel was still interviewing witnesses. The person he was talking to looked familiar. Lili placed her hand above her eyes for a better look. It was Cristina. What did she have to discuss with the FBI agent?

Lili was determined to find out.

- 14 -

OLIVER

The Secret
Wednesday, May 25, 2033, 2:30 p.m.

Oliver Stuart Robinson went up the stairs, down the hallway, and through his lab to his office. This time, he did not greet anyone. His team members briefly looked up. Sensing tension in the air, they quickly busied themselves at the benches again.

Oliver carefully closed the office glass door behind him. His office was his refuge, his sanctuary. Nothing could get to him here. Or so he thought. He sat down at his mahogany desk and took a deep breath. *What a morning!*

Now, he could finally look through the file that Ingrid had neatly placed in the middle of his desk, right in front of him. Thanks to the piles of other files around it, Lili had not noticed it, but even if she had, the uniform black cover did not reveal what was inside.

Oliver opened the file and looked with great interest through the printouts of medical images in it. The first case was a patient with a staphylococcus aureus pneumonia. The CT scan showed "tree-in-bud" opacifications. Oliver knew that these opacifications often developed due to spread of an infection through the bronchial tree, and this had been also the case in this patient, who had been exposed to bacteria via an infested air conditioner. The "tree-in-bud" opacification had been initially described in patients with tuberculosis, but it was later also described in patients with many other airborne infections, including bacterial and fungal infections. Oliver studied the images with great interest.

He turned to the next case. It was a patient who had been treated for COVID-19 and then developed pneumocystis jiroveci pneumonia. Oliver remembered that this type of pneumonia was common in patients with immunodeficiency and HIV, but this patient did not have such history. The CT scan showed bilateral ground-glass opacities and septal thickening of the lungs.

Oliver read the notes of the patient. The infection had completely resolved. This case was remarkable!

The next case was a CT scan of the chest which showed multiple snall nodules in the lung with a typical halo sign, a rim of ground-glass opacity around the nodule. Oliver remembered that these findings were usually seen in cancer patients, who had an impaired immune response after chemotherapy. But this patient had received cortisone treatment and was then exposed to the fungus through an infected facial steamer at a cosmetic studio. A follow up CT scan several months later was normal.

Oliver took some notes. Fortunately, the patients had agreed to donate leftover blood samples from their routine blood tests to research at SUEC. Oliver checked the files of these patients, and blood samples were available from all of them in the SUEC storage facility. That would make it easy to run a few tests.

He dialed the number of his patent attorney, Juri Rosen-Smith. "Hello, Juri. I received the paperwork for the patent, so I signed it and sent it back to you."

"Hello, Dr. Robinson. Yes, I received your files, and I finalized them. You confirmed that Dr. Maulvi is not a co-inventor of this work, correct? It seems that many of the submitted figures and descriptions of methods were created by her, but she simply carried out your instructions, and did not provide creative input, right?"

"Yes, correct. Dr. Maulvi and other members of my team were hired to carry out the work. They did not invent anything."

"Okay, thanks for confirming this. The patent is finalized. You can now license it or start your own company. Congratulations!"

"It's great to hear that indeed! Thanks for your help, Juri. I expect to proceed with the licensing process very soon. I was already contacted by interested parties."

"Excellent! Good luck with that!"

Oliver hung up and send a text message to Nathanael Zhang, CEO of OrchidBio, the largest up-and-coming biotech company in California. *Hello, Nathanael, patent is finalized. We are on track.*

Oliver's phone rang a minute later. It was Nathanael himself. "Hello, Oliver, this is great news! I will put in a bid tonight to license your patent."

"I'm glad to hear that. This is a unique opportunity. We will make history together!"

"Yeah, I hope so. We will have to work on acceptance by the public, though. An alliance between OrchidBio and SUEC will be crucial for that. Did you have a chance to discuss this with the university Dean, Dr. Hill? When I discussed our interest in investing in human engineering with him a few months ago, he was not very accommodating. Quite the opposite."

"I know. But I have great insider information: Dr. Hill is planning to step down."

"Wow, that could help us quite a bit. If his successor is more supportive, of course."

Oliver chuckled. "I'm quite sure he will be. But please keep this confidential for now. You should hear the official announcement soon enough."

"You have impressed me once more!"

"I am very excited about our partnership. Together, we will create humans 2.0!"

"I look forward to it. My company will invest heavily, and I look forward to generous returns!"

"You will soon be a billionaire. Take care!"

Oliver stepped towards the window. What a beautiful day today! He had always marveled at the beauty of the rainbow eucalyptus trees in front of his office. There were hundreds of varieties of the myrtle family, *myrtaceae*, but this one was exceptional. The colors of their trunks ranged among shades of green, blue, orange, red, and purple, as if someone had pained them with long strokes of multicolored crayons. They were simply magnificent.

The mission of SUEC was to select and amplify superlatives: exceptional scientists, new generations of computer algorithms, amplifications of the most stunning varieties of biological life. That was what SUEC was about. And these trees were a living monument to this noble concept. SUEC had managed to adapt the trees such that they could live in Northern California, and SUEC would adapt humans in the same manner—humans who would be stronger than any virus or bacteria on this planet.

Oliver would lead this evolutionary revolution and go into history books as the leader who created humans 2.0. The rainbow tree was his inspiration. Therefore, he had chosen a lab space that would provide him with a view of these most stunning trees in the world.

Oliver looked through the long, silvery-green leaves and clusters of tiny white flowers. On the ground below him, the FBI agent was still interviewing people. Was he talking with Cristina right now?

Oliver tried to find a good spot that provided an unobstructed view between the three branches. It was clearly her thick, perfectly ironed hair, which glistened in the sunlight. He remembered running his fingers through it and down her body. He missed that. She was classy. The most beautiful woman he had ever met.

What did Cristina have to discuss with the FBI agent? Oliver watched her from above, trying to read her gestures.

And then, to make matters worse, on the left end of the park, Lili Pham came walking towards them. What did this woman not understand about keeping her nose out of this business? He would have to discipline her. And perhaps he could help the FBI agent along in the process. That man was clearly incapable of making progress on his own.

It was very important that Nia's case would be closed before the announcement of the patent. This incident could not interfere with the publicity of their invention.

SUEC was at the dawn of a new era.

- 15 -

CRISTINA

The Confession
Wednesday, May 25, 2033, 2:30 p.m.

After the confrontation with Oliver, Cristina ran out of the building. She was upset about herself for losing her composure in front of him. But why was that her fault? He knew her vulnerabilities, and he pushed her buttons every time. *Nia's death was God's plan?*

Cristina's head was spinning. She needed to cool off. The heat outside was roasting her already fuming mind. She walked towards the adjacent park, fighting back tears. This morning had been too much. She felt so *guilty*.

In the distance, she spotted FBI agent Terrel Wright speaking with an elderly black man under a group of tall eucalyptus trees. Cristina walked towards them. She loved this place with the multi-colored trees. It was a feast for the senses. The view up the tall trees was stunning, and the air smelled like a mixture of mint and honey. It reminded her of the fragrance of the southern Peruvian Andes.

Cristina took a deep breath and then approached the two men slowly. She could not shut down the voice of her inner conscience: *Let no evil talk come out of your mouth.* She had to confess.

The FBI agent shook the hand of the other man, who turned around and disappeared behind large blooming rhododendron bushes. Agent Terrel looked at Cristina.

Let's get this over with, she thought. She summoned all of her courage and stepped towards him. "Hello, Agent Wright. Could I have a brief word?"

"Of course. What's the matter?"

"I want to make a confession." Cristina swallowed. Swelling tears blurred the man in front of her.

"What is that?" he asked.

"I cursed her. Last night." There it was. It felt good to share the burden with the FBI agent.

He looked at her. "Do you mean Nia? You 'cursed her?' What did you say to her?"

Cristina swelled. "Well, as I explained earlier, Nia was supposed to work on a very important research grant that was supported by the National Institutes of Health (NIH). In fact, this is my *only* NIH grant. There was only one researcher funded by this grant, and this was Nia. To get more NIH funding in the future, it was extremely important that we make progress. Our annual report was coming up, and Nia had not produced anything. Even worse, she used my research funds to run lab tests for some other project, for which she did not provide any results at all. What should I write in my progress report? Who did she think would pay her salary if she did not produce anything? I confronted her multiple times. She kept assuring me that results would be forthcoming. But they didn't. I was afraid that we would lose our NIH funding because of her. So, yesterday, I cursed her."

"What did you say to her?" Terrel asked again.

Cristina took a deep breath. "Well, I told her that she would be held responsible for her actions. The arc of the universe is long, but it bends towards justice! I wished from the bottom of my heart that if my career died, hers would die as well. And now, she is dead."

"So, you are afraid that you caused her death somehow?"

Cristina nodded. She reached for a Kleenex in her pocket and wiped the corners of her eyes.

"If I could just wish all criminals to prison, my work would be so much easier," Terrel said with a gentle smile.

Cristina smiled as well. "I know. It is irrational. I am a scientist and should not have such thoughts. But I grew up in a religious family. I cannot just forget all the lessons I learned as a child. And I don't want to. My faith gives me strength in this jungle of intrigue and politics. There is more evil here than in the Peruvian rainforest. And I cannot stop wondering: Did my wish bring forces into motion that we just don't understand yet?"

Terrel waved towards a bench under one of the trees. "Please sit for a moment," he said with a calm voice.

Cristina sat down and blew her nose. Terrel took a seat beside her. A small squirrel crossed in front of them.

"I think I understand some of the thoughts that might trouble you," he said. "I also grew up in a religious family. My grandmother used to say that it is a sin to wish evil on another soul. Even if they hurt you or threaten your existence, you should wish them well. Because we believe that God—or some may call it fate or karma—will bring justice upon all of us."

Cristina nodded. "That's why I am so devastated. I did wish divine justice upon her. I shouldn't have done that. I should have just terminated her contract and hired somebody else. If I had done that, perhaps she would be alive now."

"Nobody knows what would have happened. Perhaps she would have killed herself if she had lost her job. You can only reflect on the choices that you made for yourself. You cannot control other people's choices. Christians believe in the concepts of confession and forgiveness. You reflect on your deeds, you acknowledge your mistakes, and you become a better person in the process. That's what you just did."

Cristina nodded. "Thank you! That means a lot to me."

Terrel smiled. "You are welcome. Well, I have to point out that there is a fine line here. If you just had some thoughts about punishing Nia for her ignorance and disobedience and all this stayed in the world of your imagination, that's something you could discuss with your priest. However, if you actually did hurt her in our physical world, that would be my area of jurisdiction. Do you understand the difference?"

"Of course!" Cristina exclaimed. "I would never physically hurt anyone, let alone any of my team members."

Terrel nodded. "I thought so. If you didn't poison or shoot her, you did not kill Nia."

"Poison her?"

"Just figuratively speaking."

Cristina laced her hands. "I understand. I certainly did not poison or shoot her. And I sincerely hope that my curse did not harm her."

Terrel looked at her. "You're a scientist, right? So, let's do an experiment. You make a wish right now to attract justice for the murderer. We will see if it comes true. If it doesn't, you might be reassured that your dark thoughts had no influence on the real world. If your wish does come through, the killer will get caught, and you have done the FBI a great favor."

Cristina looked at Terrel, deciding what to do. He had a point here. Why not do an experiment to see if she had the power to make things happen? Some part of her thought that this was ridiculous. But another part of her did believe.

"Okay, here it comes," she said calmly. She closed her eyes and extended her arms, palms facing the sky. "*I wish that the person who killed Nia would be punished. And I wish that the person who ordered Nia's murder would feel the same pain as her parents are feeling right now.*"

"Wow, that was quite specific," Terrel said. "Do you know anything about the actual case that I don't? This would be the right time to share it with me."

Cristina shrugged. "I just expressed what I feel. From my childhood in South America, I remember that there is often a brain and a hand to a crime—and these are attached to different bodies. One person ordered Nia's murder, and another executed it. That's how most murders work. I want justice for both. The hand should be cut off. And the brain should suffer."

"Well, I certainly hope I will never cross your path! If you do find real evidence, please let me know. Remember, the justice part is up to law enforcement."

"Of course." Cristina got up from her seat. "It was really good talking with you, Agent Wright. It will be my personal penance to help find the shooter and bring them to your doorstep!" She extended her hand, and he shook it.

"Excellent! I could use any help I can get. If you see anything unusual or suspicious, please give me a call." Terrel handed her his business card.

***

Neither Cristina nor Terrel had noted Dr. Robinson behind the window or the man behind the rhododendron bushes. He had put his cell phone on recording mode and, with a long tree branch, pushed it under the bushes to the bench where the two were sitting. He waited until the two had left, then retrieved his phone.

- 16 -

LILI

The Discovery
Wednesday, May 25, 2033, 3:00 p.m.

Lili saw Cristina and Terrel talking under the trees. She walked towards them. In the distance, she saw Cristina breaking out in tears and Terrel comforting her. She stopped, trying to understand what was happening there. Some intimate conversation. It was probably better to give them some space.

Lili's stomach growled. She realized that she had not had lunch yet. During her call weeks, her schedule was completely messed up. She needed to fuel up to stay alert. More coffee. And proteins.

Lili walked over to the coffee booth and ordered a sandwich and cappuccino to go. She sat down at one of the bistro tables and gulped down the sandwich. Cheese and tomato. Delicious. She felt energized. Then she slowly strolled back.

When she arrived at the bench, Cristina and Agent Wright were gone. A man was crawling under the bench, reaching for something underneath the bushes.

"Can I help you?"

The man leaped up and bumped his head against the bench. "I'm fine, I'm fine," he mumbled. "I dropped my cell phone, but I found it." He slowly got up and waved a phone in his right hand.

Lili looked at the man. Something about him was off, but she could not quite put her finger on what it was. He had dark rings around his eyes. He looked tired, perhaps exhausted. A homeless person? No, his shirt was freshly ironed, and his face was perfectly shaved.

The man brushed the dirt of his trousers and put the cell phone into the side pocket of his jacket. Was there a grip of a gun in that same pocket? Lili stepped to the right to get a better view. As the man removed his hand from the pocket, she could see it clearly. It was a gun!

A shiver went down her spine. The man followed Lili's gaze. She looked away. He quickly closed the zipper, turned around, and left.

Lili sat down and placed her coffee mug on the bench. She grabbed her iPhone and took some photos of the man, but she only got photos of his backside as he disappeared in the park. *Should I follow him?* she thought. *No, that might be too dangerous.*

It would be better to talk with Terrel Wright. Cristina had likely returned to the research building. Or Terrel was still with her. Either way, he could decide to pick up the phone or not. She dialed his number. He did not pick up.

Lili walked back down the path that she had come earlier and found the two in front of the entrance of the research building. This time, she walked to them right away. "Hi, Terrel and Cristina!" She waved as she approached them.

Cristina looked up and waved back. Terrel's head turned towards the opposite direction, to the entrance. The sliding glass door opened, and Oliver Robinson stepped onto the front courtyard. "Hello, Agent Wright!" he greeted Terrel politely, then he turned towards Lili and Cristina with a brief nod. "Ladies."

Cristina curled her lips and walked past him into the building.

"Dr. Robinson, what can I do for you?" Terrel responded.

"I was wondering if you have any new insights regarding the shooter. The SUEC leadership is committed to finding this person as soon as possible. We are very concerned about the safety of our community members, and, of course, we cannot let a criminal destroy our reputation. SUEC represents the highest standards of integrity."

"We are still gathering information. I am afraid it is too early for updates."

"Well, I talked with our publicist this morning, and he will communicate that the FBI is investigating the case. If anybody else gets shot, the blame will come your way."

Terrel's figure straightened, and his voice became authoritative: "Dr. Robinson, the charge will come to the person who killed Nia Johnes—and anybody who assisted in the process."

Lili cleared her throat. "Perhaps I can share an observation?"

Terrel turned around to her. "Of course. What's the matter?"

"I just saw a man retrieving an iPhone underneath the bench where you and Cristina have been sitting. And when he put it in his pocket, it looked like he had a gun in his jacket. I took a picture of him." She opened her phone and showed the images to Terrel and Oliver Robinson.

As a radiologist, Lili was experienced in recognizing a trainee's ability to recognize a clue on a radiograph. There was a brief spark in their eyes when they saw something that they recognized. She saw this spark in Terrel's eyes now.

"This is just a man's back," Oliver Robinson concluded. "It could be anyone. And I do not see a gun anywhere."

"I am sure I saw the grip of a gun when he put the iPhone in his pocket," Lili insisted.

"Thank you, Lili," Terrel weighed in. "Can you please send me this photo? I take it from there." He bowed slightly towards her and Oliver Robinson and then left towards the park.

Dr. Robinson looked at Lili. "Would you please walk with me, Lili?"

"Of course."

He walked back into the building, Lili following closely. The Vice Dean did not say a word. They walked up the stairs and through the lab into his office. The eyes of the researchers in the lab followed them. Dr. Robinson closed the glass door. He did not offer her a seat. He stood in front of the glass façade of the office with a stern look on his face. Being a head shorter, Lili had to look up at him. In the background, she saw his team members gazing at their professor, absorbing the scene.

Oliver's eyes narrowed and his brow furrowed. He pointed his index finger at her. "Lili, I am really busy, and I cannot meet with you every two hours. So, we have to make this quick. I want to provide you with some immediate feedback regarding your behavior."

"My behavior?"

"I did not interact with you personally so far. But my observations today indicate that there are some issues."

Lili's heart plunged. This man held her portfolio in his hand—her future. He could nurture it or crush it. "What issues?" she managed to say.

"Well, this morning, you put both of us in danger by running towards a shooting scene. That was reckless and inconsiderate of others. Imagine the shooter had seen you and fired at my office. I could be dead now. We both could have been shot."

Lili frowned. "As I said earlier, it's not possible to see through the tinted windows. I've work here for years. I know what the windows look like from the outside," she said defensively.

"This is the other problem: You are not responsive to critiques," Dr. Robinson countered. "It seems that you are incapable of putting yourself in other people's shoes. You seem to be insensitive to the needs of others."

"Insensitive?" Hadn't she just heard this in another context this morning?

Dr. Robinson nodded. "Yes. As another example, you inappropriately declared Ingrid to be fine after she was assaulted."

Lili tried to save the situation. "I'm sorry if you misunderstood. I noted that she had only a superficial wound at her arm after she had been shot at. I was relieved that she was not seriously hurt."

Dr. Robinson lifted his index finger again. "You are a radiologist, Lili. Examining gunshot victims is not your expertise. Pretending to be an expert when you are not is quite unprofessional."

That was too much. He might accuse her of many things, but incompetency was not one of them. "I have a basic life support (BLS) certification, and I jobbed as a paramedic during medical school," Lili said coldly. "That's why I offered my help."

"See, there is it again. You cannot constructively take criticism. You talk back every time. You have practiced radiology for two decades now. Your paramedic experience is twenty years ago!"

Lili raised her voice. "The fact is that Ingrid had only a superficial wound on her arm. Fortunately!"

"You are not a forensic examiner, Lili. Or a detective. A few minutes ago, you accused a random man in the park of carrying a gun. Your photo showed neither a face nor a gun. Do you understand the consequences of false accusations? This man could sue you—and the University."

Lili was getting more and more frustrated. Dr. Robinson was twisting everything she said. "We were asked to say something if we saw something. That's what I did!" she exclaimed.

"Lili, faculty have lost their job over misrepresentations like this. At this critical point in your career, you should be much more careful. It could hurt you," he said in a low voice.

Lili felt a chill down her spine. Dr. Robinson could extend her position at SUEC or fire her. This was a direct threat.

She gave in. "Of course. I understand."

He smiled. "I am glad we are coming to an agreement here. If you have any concern about people or activities here on campus, then you will first communicate it to me. Is that clear?"

Lili nodded.

"From here, please focus on your clinical work and research. How should I represent your promotion to the SUEC committee if all you do is run around chasing imaginary suspects?"

Lili nodded again. "Certainly." She saw victory in his eyes. An unspoken laughter. The rush of power.

"I'm glad we're on the same page. I want to help you, Lili. Show us that you can represent the values of our community: Professionalism. Dedication to patient care. Medical innovation. You do share these values, don't you?"

She nodded. "Yes, I do."

He looked at her with a piercing gaze. "Prove it. Go to your lab. Your recent publication received a lot of positive publicity. The next one should be in progress. I do not want to see you anywhere near a crime scene. Is that clear?"

"Of course."

Oliver opened the glass door. About thirty heads were turned towards them. Oliver said loudly, "I am glad we understand each other. I will follow up with you, Lili." He did not shake her hand.

Lili stepped into the lab. The people there busied themselves at their desks and benches, but she saw their eyes following her as she walked through the lab. To her left, two guys grinned at her. *They like to watch me suffer because it makes them feel better about their own painful lives,* she thought. To her right, she saw a young man and a woman with pity in their eyes. That felt even more degrading. *Perhaps they'd secretly vouch for me, but don't have the guts to say anything,* Lili thought.

The tension in the room felt physically painful, and the path to the exit seemed endless. Lili's stomach tightened to a big, heavy knot. She felt nauseated, a taste of bile in her mouth. But she did not want to give this group the satisfaction of vomiting on the floor in front of them. She focused on the path in front of her. One more step, and another, and another.

There, she walked through the door—and almost ran into Jacub. He stood casually in the shadows of the hallway, leaning against a marble infinity statue. "Hello, professor, are you having a bad day?" He smiled at her.

Lili sighed. "I don't want to talk about it."

He walked with her, hands in his pockets. "You know, I'm your friend, Lili. Always."

Lili looked at his calm emerald-green eyes. Jacub was the most well-mannered, decent guy around here. The kind of guy who would open the door for you and walk on the more dangerous side of the sidewalk to keep you safe. "I guess I am always doing the wrong thing."

Jacub shook his head. "Criticizing others is a sport here, Lili. If someone criticizes you, the chance is high that they just have some political agenda. It has nothing to do with your worthiness. *You* know when you did the right thing. You just know it. You don't need anybody else to validate your thoughts or actions."

Lili swallowed. The knot in her stomach felt a little less painful. "Thank you!" she said.

"Any time." Jacub smiled. "By the way, did you find out what the PCR results meant?"

Lili hit her forehead with a flat palm. "I completely forgot about that. I got carried away by all of these distractions. Thanks for reminding me, Jacub. I will discuss the matter with Cristina."

"Great. Please keep me posted."

"You can come with me right now."

"As I said, please keep my name out of this. I would have to explain how I got the results. That could get me in trouble."

"Of course, I understand. I'll let you know what I find out."

"Thanks! And don't ever lose your no-nonsense spirit, Lili. That's what many of us love and respect about you." He bowed slightly towards her, turned around, and went down the stairs.

Lili watched his disappearing silhouette. *Sometimes, all you need is just one person who validates the core of your being,* she thought.

Lili walked down the hallway to Cristina's office. She knocked at the door. There was a ruffling noise, and then Cristina's voice answered. "Come in!"

She stuck her head through the door: "Hello, Cristina, are you busy?"

Cristina sat at her desk, looking at her with one mascara-smudged eye and one mascara-cleaned eye. Lili couldn't help but smile. "Sorry, I didn't mean to interrupt."

Cristina shook her head. "No worries. Please come in. I won't get much done today, anyways. I'm still processing Nia's death."

Lili stepped into the room and closed the door behind her. "Well, that's why I'm here as well. I got some results from a PCR analysis that apparently Nia had been doing recently. I'm not sure what I'm looking at. Would you mind reviewing these results?"

"Of course!" Cristina responded. "How did you get these?"

"I found them in the trash can."

"Lili, you are an outstanding radiologist, but you are a terrible liar. If you found these in the trash can, how do you know these are Nia's?"

"Well, it could have been Nia's trash can. But you are right: someone handed them to me and asked me not to mention their name."

Cristina looked at her, shaking her head. "Lili, you do not toy with honesty."

"Sorry. It was a white lie to get you started here."

"There are no white lies, Lili. You know that. All lies have consequences. But let me have a look."

Lili showed Cristina the files on her iPhone. She flipped through them, then waved at the seat in front of her. "Why don't you have a seat? This will take a little while."

Cristina started examining the files on Lili's phone. She took a pen out of a drawer and made some notes. Meanwhile, Lili made herself comfortable. Since Cristina had her phone, she could not even check her emails. Her mailbox was probably overflowing right now, but there was nothing she could do about it.

The last night had been really stressful. The upper part of the seat could be turned backwards, and Lili leaned back. It only took a couple of minutes until she fell asleep.

Someone shook her shoulders. "Hey, Lili, wake up!"

She opened her eyes and saw Christina right in front of her. "Lili. I made some very interesting discoveries here. You have to see this!" She held the iPhone in front of Lili and pointed at some graphics and numbers.

Lili sat up. "What did you find?"

"Well, I would have certainly liked to examine the samples by myself, but as far as I can see from the results here, it looks like Nia, Ingrid, and five others examined here are all related—they share common genes."

"Do you mean they are genetically related? They are siblings?"

"Well, there's also some genetic inhomogeneity here, so, presumably, these individuals have different mothers, but the same father."

"Nia and Ingrid are siblings? Do you think Ingrid knows about that?"

"I don't know. But here is the real bummer: all of these individuals also share the same key genes with Oliver Robinson!"

"He is a sibling, too?"

"Considering the age difference and his birth date, I don't think he's their sibling. He is their father."

"Father? But Nia's parents arrived here this morning. She already has a father."

"I obviously don't know the circumstances, and I am not an expert in this area at all. But here's what I know: many couples nowadays use *in vitro* fertilization to conceive a baby. For one reason or another, it can make sense to use a donor for either the egg or sperm. Perhaps Oliver had an affair with all mothers of these listed siblings. This is entirely possible, considering his narcissistic character. But I googled these women, and I don't think they were his type."

Lili looked at her. "I learned from Jacub that you know a thing or two about that."

Cristina made a waving gesture. "I don't want to talk about it. Anyways, another, more plausible explanation is that he donated his sperm as a young man, and that multiple children were conceived by that, including Nia and Ingrid. It would fit his grandiose personality perfectly well, imagining that he tried to conceive as many children as possible through these means."

Lili looked at her. "Wow. Is that even legal?"

"As long as the mothers chose him as a donor without coercion from his side, it is within the law, as far as I know."

"Okay. So, let's assume for a moment that Nia and Ingrid are Dr. Robinson's daughters. How did they get to work here? Do you think they knew this before they applied for their research jobs?"

Cristina shrugged. "Nia cannot tell us anymore. But perhaps Ingrid can."

Lili shook her head. "I'm not sure about that. She didn't seem cooperative when I tried to get information from her."

"Perhaps Nia and Ingrid approached Oliver with some kind of a demand, and that got them killed—or shot at?"

"Do you think he can be violent?"

"I don't think he killed them personally. Oliver is completely self-absorbed, and I'm sure he has no scruples about removing anyone in his way. But he's also a chicken. His weapon is politics, not physical assault. If he wanted to get somebody out of the way, he would let someone else do the dirty work."

"Well, somebody is running around killing people. And I'm pretty certain we uncovered a key finding here. I think we should share this information with Agent Wright."

Cristina nodded. "Just be careful."

- 17 -

JACUB

The Gun
Wednesday, May 25, 2033, 4:00 p.m.

Jacub hummed as he walked down the stairs to the entrance hall of the research building. The student's death was a tragedy. But it had sparked his side gig. He had to run multiple errands today for SUEC researchers and the security team. People were on edge, and they were generously tipping. He had probably made a couple hundred dollars today. Not bad.

And he had helped Cristina and her friend Lili. The two women would always get his services free of charge—unless they tipped spontaneously, of course. They liked and respected him. Not like the other professors who treated him like shit—or, worse, as if he did not exist at all. Like he was air. Cristina and Lili were kind and generous. They genuinely liked him. It was a pity that they had to constantly deal with inflated egos and politics.

But he would keep them safe. He would be their protector. And perhaps one day, Cristina would see his qualities.

Jacub had never seen that husband of hers. What a lucky guy. But did he treat her as she deserved? Cristina had attended many local events at SUEC, but the husband had never joined her. He was the CEO of some company in Silicon Valley. Perhaps he was just incredibly busy. Or the two were estranged. They did not have children. And she'd had an affair with the professor. People here got divorced all the time. And when that happened, Jacub would be right there.

Dr. Robinson violated every moral value that Cristina believed in. He was perhaps a temporary toy boy. But he had no chance to keep her in the long run. He, Jacub, understood her much better. He shared her sense of honesty and moral integrity. Jacub imagined being in Dr.

Robinson's place when he kissed Cristina and she kissed him back so passionately.

"Hello, Jacub, could I have a word?"

Puzzled, Jacub looked at the FBI agent in front of him. Where had he come from? "Hello, Agent Wright. Of course, how can I be of assistance?"

"Could we go to someplace quiet? Do you have an office?"

"Of course. Come this way."

Jacub led the FBI agent down the hall and into his office, then settled on the couch and waved at the seat in front of him.

The agent looked around, then sat down. There were piles of papers and folders on Jacub's desk. A seating area more reminiscent of a living room than a manager's office. A half-finished drink was on the coffee table, and there was some yellow stain on the carpet. "This is quite a relaxed setting for a manager's office," Terrel said.

"Well, few people need a meeting to inform me about whatever issues they need fixed, and for formal meetings, we do have a conference room next door. This here is mostly for my own comfort."

Terrel pointed at the sofa on which Jacub was sitting. "Is that a sleeper sofa?"

"Yes, it is. I just thought it would be convenient in case I had to stay late at night."

"Why would you have to stay late?"

"I like to take on extra tasks if they are paid. I'm saving money to buy my own home. So, I run errands, I assist researchers with their work, and I help out at local events."

"How often do you stay late for these activities?"

"Well, I don't really keep a book on that. I do not have a family, so I'm flexible. If the payment is good, I am available."

"Did you work late on Tuesday night?"

"Let me think. I did run a lot of errands that day."

"So, you were here on Tuesday night? Until what time?"

"I don't recall off the top of my head."

Terrel make a note in his notebook, then looked up at Jacub. "Jacub, I want to share results from our forensic team with you. You mentioned that you had delivered toothpaste to Nia on the evening when she was killed?"

"Yes, correct."

"You said that she sent you an email to get a toothpaste from the grocery store next door, but when you delivered it, she was surprised?"

"Yes, that's what I said."

"Where exactly did you purchase that toothpaste?"

"In the store a few hundred meters down the street, to the left of this building."

"And you brought it to Nia directly from the store?"

"No—when I came back from the store, I received a call from Dr. Robinson that there was a problem with the freezer in the basement, so I left the toothpaste on my desk here and went down to have a look. It was one of these annoying problems. Somebody had unplugged it. So, I plugged it back in and checked that everything was okay, then went up to my office."

"Was Dr. Robinson in the basement as well when you got there?"

"No, he is far too busy. And what is he going to do? Hand me a screwdriver? No, he usually just leaves me a message about equipment that doesn't work. Most of the time, it's a trivial problem. I often wondered why such a smart man has such limited practical skills. I guess he's always had a butler."

"And what happened after you got back to your office?"

"I fetched the toothpaste tube and brought it to Nia. Why is the FBI interested in toothpaste?"

"The toothpaste was spiked with high quantities of ketamine, a very powerful anesthetic."

Jacub stared at Terrel with wide-open eyes. "You mean the toothpaste that I brought to her?"

"Yes. We found your fingerprints on it."

"I don't understand."

"Me neither. Enlighten me."

"Why would I tell you about it if I wanted to poison Nia with it? I did not put anything into her toothpaste!"

"I understand your frustration. But the evidence speaks against you. Do you have any idea who could've done this if it was not you? Who would have had access to your office?"

"I really don't know! My door is always open. Anybody can walk in here."

"Would you mind if I have a quick look around?" Terrel asked.

"Of course, be my guest! I have nothing to hide!"

The FBI agent got up from his seat and walked towards the desk on their right. There was a refrigerator in the back. He opened it. There were various food items, sodas, beer, milk, mustard, and ketchup. On the upper rack was a toothbrush and toothpaste. He took out the toothpaste and put it into an evidence bag.

"I like to clean my teeth after I eat something," Jacub explained. "I have no other place to put it."

"Of course. This is just our routine. I have to examine it to confirm that it is just regular toothpaste."

"That's what you will find!" Jacub cleaned his forehead with a paper towel. He was horrified that Nia was dead because of something he did—not with intention, but still…

Terrel continued his rounds through the room. He examined the bookshelves and found the photo of Cristina and Jacub at the SUEC reception for junior faculty that Jacub had placed between the books. Terrel opened the small wardrobe and flipped through the selection of suits and casual attire. He opened the small cabinet with the bedsheets and pillows for the night. He did not comment on any of these. He went back to the desk and looked through a stack of files on it. He pulled out a black folder with an SUEC sign.

Jacub got up from the couch to have a better look. *Where did that folder come from?* "That is not mine," he said.

"Well, it's on your desk," Terrel responded.

"I don't know how it got there. What is in it?"

Terrel opened the folder and pulled out several printouts of medical imaging studies.

The first one was a CT scan of a nine-year-old child. An attached Word file included the medical record number, the age of the patient, the clinical diagnosis, and a brief note: *Typhlitis/ neutropenic colitis in a child with leukemia and neutropenia. The images show marked bowel wall thickening of the cecum and ascending colon. Large areas of low attenuation indicate bowel wall edema. There is fat stranding around the affected bowel and free fluid.*

Terrel looked at the next case, which was labeled as: *18-year-old patient with leukemia and candida infection.* He remembered that candida albicans was the most common fungal infection in immuno-compromised patients. The images had a note: *MRI scans shows multiple lesions in the liver and spleen which demonstrate ring-like peripheral contrast enhancement, consistent with an abscess.* The lesions had been marked with arrows.

Terrel placed the images into another evidence bag. He would contact Dr. Lili Pham for confirmation of the findings described in the notes.

Jacub watched him over his shoulder. "These images are not mine!"

"I made a note of that statement, Jacub. We will investigate them for fingerprints."

Jacub felt a shiver down his spine. He had no idea where these images had come from. Someone was clearly setting him up here. "If I had known that there was anything compromising in my office, I would not have invited you to search it. I would have asked you to come back with a search warrant and removed these images in the meantime. I am being framed!"

The FBI agent looked at him and said calmly, "Jacub, this is not my first rodeo. For now, I am just collecting evidence."

He continued to look through the room, now inspecting the sofa, ottoman, and seats in front of it. Was there a small black item under the sofa?

Agent Wright got down on his knees and looked under the sofa. Jacub felt dizzy. He was pretty sure that he had not placed anything there. Whatever it was, this couldn't be good for him. He slowly stepped backwards towards the door.

Agent Wright turned the flashlight of his iPhone on and reached for the dark item. He fetched it and got back up. Jacub stared at the agent with wide-open eyes.

Terrel held a gun in his hand.

Jacub turned around and ran as fast as his feet would take him. He raced through the lobby and towards the main entrance of the building. The double glass door was coming closer. He heard the FBI agent running after him, shouting into his cell phone, "Subject on the run, south entrance of SUEC building!"

Jacub fetched the ID around his neck and made a quick turn to the right, racing towards the entrance of the imaging lab. He placed his ID on the scanner in front of the door, and the solid steel security door flung open. He jumped through and smashed it shut a split second before the FBI agent reached it. They could see each other through the small lead window in the door.

"Jacub, don't make a mistake that you'll regret later," Terrel shouted from the other side of the door. "If you are innocent, then the evidence will prove it."

"I am innocent," Jacub responded. "But unfortunately, I have not had such a favorable experience with the justice system. The powerful win, and the others loose. That's how the system works. So, I have to save myself."

He turned around. Lili was sitting with a student at the MRI scanner. They both stared at him. "What's going on?" Lili asked. From her place, she could not see the person behind the door. The MRI scanner was making so much noise that they couldn't hear much of the conversation, either.

"Just a misunderstanding," Jacub shouted back. "Dr. Robinson. Can you please wait a few minutes until you open the door?"

"It would be my great pleasure!" Lili smiled.

Jacub walked through the lab towards the back end of the building. He opened the door and stepped onto the small path behind the building. He knew the area around the building by heart. He lived here. He walked quickly along the limestone wall of the octagonal building, concealed by the shadows of the roof. Security guards were coming from the streets, running towards the main entrance, and distributing to the right and left. One of them followed Jacub's path, but he was looking towards the park, and had not spotted him yet. There were cameras all around the building, but it would take some time to review all the footage.

Jacub had reached his office. The window was still open. He reached for the window frame and quickly pulled himself inside. He threw his blazer on the sofa, jumped to the wardrobe, grabbed a black hoodie with a big SUEC label, and put it on. Perhaps this would distract the search team if they had been told to look for a man in a silver blazer.

He cowered under the desk as he saw Terrel running by the window, but Terrel did not see him. Jacub was breathing heavily from his sprint, and he tried to catch his breath now. His chest hurt, and sweat was running down his temples. *Breathe*, he thought. *Think*. He had survived worse. But he could not stay here for long. Since the FBI agent had found a gun here, he would surely be back.

Jacub opened the top drawer of his desk and removed an FOB key. He peeked towards the window. No more people running by. Perhaps this was a good time.

He got up and walked through the hallway towards a small conference room on the West side of the building, which was just a few meters away from the grocery store. Fortunately, the conference room was empty. Jacub quickly slipped in, closed the door, and walked past the large conference table and scattered chairs to a large window at the back end of the room.

A few meters away, several small electric vehicles were standing on a small parking lot. These were used to deliver goods to the buildings on campus, and Jacub had received authorization to use them for his errands.

He looked around. There was a security guard to his right. He looked towards the street, grabbed the plastic trash can beside the table, opened the door carefully, avoiding any noise, and jumped through. He slowly walked towards the electric vehicles, holding the trash can with both arms, as if it were very heavy, and hiding his face behind it. The security guard turned around, looked at him briefly, and turned back towards the street.

Jacub had reached the cars. He opened the door of the car closest to him, got in, placed the trashcan on the passenger seat, started the engine, and slowly drove down the street. He wanted to turn right to exit the campus but saw a police car close to the campus entrance, so he turned left and drove up the hill. Perhaps he could escape through the forest.

It was rare that electric vehicles would drive up to the main administrative building. The promenade was mostly used by walkers and bikers. There were many of them on the street, and they did not try to make space for the vehicle. Jacub tried to control his impatience as he slowly maneuvered around them.

Suddenly, he saw another vehicle approaching in the rearview mirror—an SUEC security vehicle. They were coming for him!

Jacub hit the accelerator and raced up the promenade. Screaming and shouting pedestrians were jumping out of his way. The vehicle behind him accelerated as well. Was that the FBI agent behind the wheel? How had he found him?

Jacub had reached the upper part of the promenade. To his left was a steep hillside, and to his right was dense forest. In front of him was the terrace of the administrative building of the university. It was only a few meters to the forest behind it.

As he reached the terrace, he yanked the wheel to the right. There was the coffee booth. He hit the brakes. He saw the wide-open eyes of the barista, who jumped out of the booth two seconds before his car smashed into it. The car bounced off to the right, and the scenery behind the front window took a 360-degree turn. Then, it hit the ground.

Jacub felt the smash, then a dull pain on his chest. The airbags had deployed. He felt dizzy. It smelled like fire.

The passenger door of the car was opened, and someone released the seatbelt, grabbed his arms, and pulled him out of the car. He saw Terrel's face in front of him. "Jacub Bezdomny, you are under arrest."

Then, he lost consciousness.

- 18 -

HEINZ

The Sandwich
Wednesday, May 25, 2033, 4:00 p.m.

Heinz had retreated to his office in order to complete a number of tasks that he had received from his manager, Atharv Patel. They were both working for the IT team at SUEC, Heinz mostly remotely, Atharv largely onsite at the University campus. They had only met twice in person, first for Heinz's job interview and next at the inauguration of Atharv's husband as Dean of the University. Apart from that, Heinz and Atharv largely communicated via email or Zoom. That worked perfectly for both of them.

Atharv was very outgoing. He loved personal interactions with clients, while Heinz preferred the serenity of his home office. Ever since he was a child, Heinz loved to be home. It reminded him of those precious moments when he would play with his dog in the backyard— a different dog at the time—and his mom would cook his favorite meal.

Heinz didn't miss office politics, and he definitely did not miss cubicles. These were simply a terrible way to work. His commute was the length of the hallway, he could arrange his desk as he wanted, and he did not have to share it with anyone. He did not have to dress up and was comfortable all day long.

Heinz adjusted the photo of Nia, Ingrid, and him on his desk. Apart from Atharv, Nia, and Ingrid were the first real live friends he'd had in a very long time. In fact, Nia and Ingrid were more. They were family. Except Nia was dead now.

Heinz got up from his desk and walked over to the guest room, where Ingrid was taking a nap. The door was ajar, and he peeked through the small gap. She was lying on the bedspread, her head resting on a pillow, a thin wool blanket covering her gracile body. Her eyes were closed, and her chest was slowly moving up and down. She was sleeping. Her silky long hair outlined the perfectly symmetric features of her face—the incarnation of youthful beauty, lulled in peaceful silence.

Heinz felt an overwhelming urge to protect her, to keep her safe from whoever wanted to harm her. He wished he had a superpower, the power to protect her, like Superman, a man who could save people. But he was just a regular guy. What would he do if an intruder came into this house? He didn't have a gun. He was big, but he was not particularly strong, and he was tired himself.

He closed the door quietly, carefully avoiding any noise. Then he tiptoed back to his office.

Schnitzel hadn't cared to join him on his excursion to the guest room. That was unusual. He liked to follow Heinz from one room to another, always looking for an opportunity to fetch a treat or go for a walk. Why could the pooch not warm up to Ingrid? Perhaps he sensed that he would have to share Heinz with her, and wasn't ready for it.

Heinz looked at his beloved dog. Schnitzel was lying under the desk, weeping, as if he'd had a bad dream. He patted the dog's head. "You will always be my favorite furball," he whispered. The dog opened his eyes. They looked watery. Was he sick?

Heinz felt a little beside himself as well, but he really had to get this work done. He sat down at his desk and tried to focus on the computer screen, but he could not stop thinking about Nia and Ingrid. Why had Nia brought him the laptop? What was so interesting about it?

He fetched the laptop from the drawer and opened it. The list of medical cases appeared again. What did these files mean? What was so important about them that some maniac would kill for it? There had to be a pattern that connected them all. Perhaps he just had to review a few more to understand it.

Heinz randomly opened one of the files. The bones were bright, so this was a CT scan. The notes stated that it was a CT scan of the abdomen of a patient with pyelonephritis, an infection of the kidneys. The patient had presented with high fever and flank pain. The CT scan had been obtained after intravenous contrast injection. The kidneys showed wedge-shaped areas of reduced contrast enhancement. The notes stated that the patient had been treated with antibiotics and had completely recovered.

Heinz opened another case, labeled as emphysematous pyelonephritis, an acute severe necrotizing infection of the kidney. The notes stated that the CT scan showed rim-enhancing abscesses in the left kidney. One of the abscesses contained air, which was indicative of the disease. The notes also stated that this patient had diabetes, a predisposing condition, and that these infections usually were very severe, but fortunately, the patient recovered completely.

What was the pattern here? What did all these images have in common? Heinz could not wrap his head around it. All the images showed infections, but they were in different locations. Some were in the brain, others in the lungs, abdomen, or pelvis. It wasn't about the type of infection, either. Some were caused by viruses, others by bacteria or fungi.

Heinz opened a third case, labeled as a CT scan of a child with hemolytic uremic syndrome. The notes stated that the disease was caused by *E. coli* bacteria, which the patient had likely ingested with contaminated food. The bacteria colonized the colon and infiltrated of the bowel wall. From there, the bacteria penetrated vessels, circulated in the blood, and caused a renal failure. The CT scan showed a marked swelling and hemorrhage of the colon and kidneys.

Heinz felt a little nauseated as well. Perhaps he had caught some infection as well. He had difficulty focusing on the text in front of him. His vision blurred, and the letters started to dance around in front of his eyes.

Heinz wiped his forehead with the back of his hand. The events this morning had been too much. He wasn't used to stress like this. First the message about Nia's death, then Ingrid at his doorstep, escaping a shooter.

He felt completely overwhelmed. How should he keep Ingrid safe? He did not want to lose another sister. He longed to have a family again.

But he was not brave. He was scared. He did not have anything here to defend them.

It was too much. He felt exhausted and scared.

And then his mind slowly drifted away.

- 19 -

TERREL

The Threat
Wednesday, May 25, 2033, 4:30 p.m.

FBI agent Terrel Wright walked into the lobby of the SUEC administrative building at the top of the hill. He had handed Jacub over to his FBI colleagues, who had taken the man into custody. Jacub had continued to plead that he was innocent and that someone had framed him.

The evidence would shed light on that.

Terrel opened the heavy entrance door of the SUEC building and stepped into the lobby. This time, Dr. Hill's administrative associate, Aiko Tanaka, greeted him at the reception. Terrel remembered her fondly. She had helped him to arrest a criminal last year. It was rare to meet a receptionist who was also a fifth-degree black belt holder.

"Great to see you again, Aiko," he said.

"Hello, Agent Wright! Always at your service," she responded with a broad smile. "When you come visit us, trouble is around. I just saw your colleagues arresting our building manager. He is an honest, hardworking guy. I cannot believe he committed any crime."

"We are in the middle of our investigation. If he is innocent, then we'll clear him soon."

"I hope so. Did you want to meet Dr. Hill?"

"Yes, that's why I'm here."

"He has no visitors at the moment, so you can directly go up and see him if you like. He asked me to reschedule all non-urgent meetings today and tomorrow."

"Why did he do that?"

"I guess he wanted to keep his calendar free in case any meetings came up to discuss the death of the SUEC student. Poor man. The incident has hit him hard. He's not quite himself. He seems very distracted and very depressed."

"I'm sorry to hear that. It must've been quite a shock. Our team is certainly working hard to solve this case as quickly as possible and bring the shooter to justice."

Aiko nodded. She waved him to the iris scanner and through the metal detector. The computer cleared him with a *beep*. "You're good to go. You know the way to his office, right?"

Terrel nodded. "Yes, I do. No worries."

He walked through the diamond-shaped atrium towards the steel column in the center, which rose three stories high to the gigantic octagonal cupola on the top. The sun sent golden rays through the prismatic glass of the cupola, creating multicolored sparkles around him. Light piano music played in the background—Chopin. A humanoid robot with a coffee tray passed by and disappeared in an elevator inside the central column. The base of the central pillar was lined by an indoor garden of potted orchid plants. Terrel walked past the beautiful flowers and up the spiral glass stairway to the second floor. Two students came down the hallway, chatting with each other. Terrel knocked on Dr. Hill's office.

"Come in."

Dean Hill sat at his desk, his face pale, dark circles under his hollow eyes.

"Hello, Dr. Hill. I hope I'm not interrupting anything?"

"Not at all. I am only writing my resignation letter." Robert Hill pointed at the computer screen in front of him.

"I hope it doesn't come to that."

"Well, I cannot imagine how all of my problems would be solved in the next twenty-four hours."

"Perhaps not all of them, but the one that involved a hired stripper."

Roberts eyes widened. "A hired stripper?"

"Yeah. Based on your descriptions and the photo that you forwarded to me, we checked the footage of the security cameras of the hotel where you stayed. We got a pretty good head shot of your Adonis—"

"It is not 'my Adonis!'"

"—of course not. Anyways, we found him. From there, it took some time to track down the original client. She used an alias and several middlemen. It was Dr. Ingrid Maulvi."

"I'm sorry, who is that?"

"She's the lab manager in Dr. Oliver Robinson's lab."

"Wow! Do you think Dr. Robinson is behind this? He's the Vice Dean at SUEC. He would take my place if I were to step down."

"I told you it was politics. I can hand over the information to your security team if you'd like. However, we only have evidence that the lab manager was involved in the case. We do not have any evidence that Dr. Robinson even knew about any of this. If he gave the order, he covered his tracks."

"And he would likely find a way to send the compromising images to my husband, regardless of what we do with the manager."

"That is a possibility."

The Dean shook his head. "It cannot happen. I'd rather step down."

"And hand over all the power of your position to somebody with questionable integrity?"

"I know. It's an impossible situation. Perhaps I could just announce another candidate."

"From what I understand, Dr. Robinson has worked for years as your second hand, and is member of the SUEC Board. It will be very difficult to appoint another successor. And even if you managed that, that person would likely be blackmailed as well."

"You are correct. We are in an impossible situation."

"Can you not just talk with your husband?"

"Atharv cannot see these photos. It would ruin our relationship, and our planned adoption. I just know it. And imagine if the photos circulated more widely. We have many conservative donors and board members. It is already hard for them to bear that the SUEC Dean is gay. A gay cheating scandal would be too much for them—I would surely have to step down. So, better to do it now. Hopefully, this will prevent my total embarrassment and the destruction of everything that is dear to me."

Terrel nodded. "Of course, I understand. You were asked to step down by tomorrow. Give me these twenty-four hours. This incident has to be connected with Nia's death somehow. It would be too much of a coincidence for these events to happen on the same day."

"I don't see how these could be connected."

"Well, for starters, Dr. Ingrid Maulvi, the lab manager, was also shot at this morning."

"Oh, this is the woman who was assaulted on campus today? I didn't realize that it was the same person."

"Yes, indeed. I did talk with her briefly after the incident. She was unusually composed. Dr. Segond examined her at the hospital, and she wondered if the wound on her arm was self-inflicted."

"Self-inflicted?"

"This is only an assumption. Our forensic team is examining the evidence at this time. But, considering what we just learned, I definitely need to talk with her again. I will ask my colleagues to find her."

Dr. Hill's desk phone rang. "Excuse me." He picked it up. "Yes, of course. Please send her up."

He hung up and looked at Terrel. "Dr. Lili Pham is here. She wants to talk with us."

"Interesting. Lili is an excellent detective. I wonder what she's found." Terrel grabbed two chairs from the adjacent conference table and placed them in front of the desk. He sat down on one. "It looks like this will take a bit longer than I had anticipated."

"Be my guest," Robert Hill said.

Someone knocked at the door. "Come in," Dr. Hill shouted.

Lili opened the door. "Hello, do you have a minute?"

"Of course! Did you come to see me or Agent Wright?"

"Both." Lili came in and sat down on the vacant chair. "I know your time is precious. Let me cut right to the chase." She pulled up her cell phone and handed it to Terrel.

Terrel looked at the screen. "What is this?" he asked.

"These are PCR tests of blood samples of several people we know: Nia, Ingrid, and Dr. Robinson. There's also an analysis of a blood sample of a Heinz Tremblay. I don't know him, but I googled him, and it seems that he works for our university IT team. "

"And what do the PCR analyses show?" Terrel asked.

"Well, as you know, I am a radiologist. I do not work with PCRs. I reviewed these with Cristina. We found something quite surprising, and I came here so that you could check if our interpretation is accurate."

"And what is that?" Dean Hill asked.

"It seems that Nia, Ingrid, and Heinz are half-siblings."

"Half-siblings?"

"Meaning that they have one parent in common. But what is even more interesting is that all three are related to Dr. Robinson."

"Dr. Robinson is their brother?"

"More likely their father."

Dean Hill shook his head. "Dr. Robinson has two children in their early twenties, a boy and a girl, and these people here are not either of them."

Lili nodded. "These are additional children."

Dean Hill looked at her. "From an affair?"

"The three have three different mothers."

"Wow," said Dr. Hill. "No wonder he wants to frame others for affairs. He seems to have a lot of experience with those."

Lili looked at them with raised eyebrows. "Dr. Robinson frames others for having affairs?"

"That's a different story," said Dr. Hill.

Terrel looked at her. "That's an interesting discovery."

Lili nodded. "I know it sounds quite fantastic. But with your resources, you could check if this is, in fact, true. Imagine these children somehow found out that their father was a wealthy, world-famous professor. Perhaps they threatened him somehow…"

"That's quite an allegation," Terrel said. "Where did you get these PCR analyses?"

"I can't say."

"Lili, we are investigating a homicide. More people could get killed," Terrel said.

"You could get killed," Robert Hill added.

Lili looked from one man to the other. "Can you please keep this confidential? I promised to not tell anyone."

"Of course!"

Lili sighed. "Jacub found these in the PCR machine in our research building and took photos of them. Perhaps that's why someone planted a gun in his office."

"We don't know that yet," Terrel said. "Our forensic team is investigating the evidence."

"Is it possible to plant fingerprints on a gun?" Lili asked.

"Yeah, one can create latex copies of someone's fingerprints with CAD/CAM software and place the prints on an object. But prints alone are not enough to prosecute someone. We need more evidence to put them at the scene, and we will certainly investigate the evidence very carefully. Can you please forward these PCR files to me? Our team will check them out."

Lili's thumbs flew over her phone. Two seconds later, Terrel found the files in his mailbox. "Got them, thank you!" He sent the files to his forensic team and asked them to analyze them. He also asked them to locate Dr. Ingrid Maulvi.

"Thank you, Lili. You've provided important evidence for our investigation."

"I'm glad I could help. I really hope that we find the murderer soon."

"We are doing everything we can to make that happen. I'm afraid I have to leave now."

Terrel nodded towards Lili and Dean Hill. Then, he left Dr. Hill's office, walked back down to the entrance hall, and left the SUEC building. He crossed the terrace in front of the building. The SUEC security team was busy cleaning up the mess from Jacub's accident earlier today. A group of students was taking photos of the smashed coffee booth.

Terrel walked past them and down the promenade. It was hot. He took off his jacket. The cell phone rang. He tried to untangle his arm from the jacket to pick up the phone. It was one of his team members. "Hi, Terrel. We found an unresponsive man in a single-family home in San Francisco. He seems to be an SUEC employee— Heinz Tremblay."

Terrel couldn't believe his ears. That was the same man they had just talked about. "I'm on my way. Call an ambulance. They should bring him to SUEC hospital. Request an exam by Dr. Annya Segond."

- 20 -

HEINZ

The K-Hole
Wednesday, May 25, 2033, 5:00 p.m.

Heinz felt as if he were rising above his body and watching himself from afar. Like a near-death experience. His body had slipped from his desk chair and was lying on the floor of his San Francisco home. His limbs felt far away, numb. He couldn't move or speak.

He saw Schnitzel lying beside him. The dog's head was resting on his chest, eyes closed. Heinz was not sure if Schnitzel was alive or dead. He felt panic tightening his throat. He wanted to scream for help, but his tongue was frozen.

An angel stepped into the room, fetched the dog, and carried him out of the room. Where were they going? Schnitzel never left his side.

Heinz wanted to jump up and follow them. But he could not move.

A wave of despair washed over him. He was paralyzed, his body trapped in a silent scream.

He had failed to protect his best friend.

He wasn't sure how long he had been in this helpless, frozen state. He tried to move, but he could not.

After what seemed to be an eternity, Heinz heard steps coming down the hallway. A female police officer was kneeling down beside him, feeling the pulse at his neck. She made a phone call. A few minutes later, he heard the sirens of an ambulance arrive. Two paramedics came running into the room. They examined his body, fixed an oxygen cannula on his nose, and placed an intravenous line. Then, they put him on a stretcher and carried him down the stairs, through the hallway on the first floor, through the door, and into the back cabin of the ambulance. The oxygen must have done something, because Heinz could move his eyes and eyelids again.

The paramedics stepped aside, and a black man with short dreadlocks looked at him. "Hello, Mr. Tremblay. My name is Terrel Wright; I am a special agent for the FBI. If you can understand me, can you please close your eyes?"

Heinz tried to move his eyelids. They were so heavy. He could not move them. He stared at the agent.

"If you can understand me, can you please close your eyes?" the agent repeated.

Heinz thought of Schnitzel. Where was he? Who had taken him away? Was Ingrid hurt? He summoned all of his strength and closed his eyes.

"Excellent. We have a mode of communication. If you want to say yes, close your eyes like that. If you want to say no, close and open your eyes twice. Do you understand?"

Heinz closed his eyes again. It got easier with practice.

"Thank you. Did you try to kill yourself today?"

Heinz tried to concentrate on his eyes. Close and open, close and open. It was difficult to move them so many times. They felt so heavy.

"Did you take drugs today?"

Close and open, close and open.

"Did someone poison you?

Close.

"Do you know which drug they gave you?"

Close and open, close and open.

"Was somebody else in your home?"

Close.

"A man?"

Close and open, close and open.

"A woman?"

Close.

"A child?"

Close and open, close and open.

"A pet?"

Close.

Heinz had run out of energy. He could not lift his eyelids again.

"Mr. Tremblay, can you hear me?"

Heinz tried. But he could not find the strength to open his eyes again.

"Okay, we'll bring you to the hospital now and make sure that you feel better soon. In the meantime, I will have a look at your home to see if I find anything unusual. I will also look for the woman and the pet. There is nobody here besides you. Do you have photos of them in the house?"

Heinz's eyes opened wide. He closed them. The heart monitor beeped to signal an increased heart rate. He opened his mouth and tried to speak. "Schnnnn." His voice gave in.

"Okay, Mr. Tremblay. Don't worry, we'll find them. I will come to see you in the hospital later today."

Heinz tried to tell the man Schnitzel's name again. But his tongue was petrified. He wanted to scream, "My dog is in danger!" But he could not move his tongue.

The man left. The paramedics jumped into the ambulance, the doors shut, the siren turned on, and the ambulance raced down the street.

Heinz must have dozed off. When he opened his eyes again, he found himself in a hospital bed. The black man was standing beside him, talking with a very attractive middle-aged redhead in a white coat.

"Most criminals use the same *modus operandi*," the woman said. "Nia was drugged with ketamine. Assuming that the same drug was used here, Mr. Tremblay likely experienced a K-hole."

"What is that?" the man asked.

"Ketamine blocks glutamate, a neurotransmitter in the brain. This blocks signaling pathways between the conscious mind and other parts of your brain. It can cause a dissociative feeling of being separate from one's own body—a frightening experience that can lead to panic attacks. Our patient here had these as well. He still has a high heartrate and high blood pressure. He is distressed about something."

"Will the paralysis go away?"

"Yes, the toxic effects of ketamine are typically short-lived. He should be able to move and speak again shortly."

"Okay. I'll stay with him and wait for that to happen."

"Sounds good. I have to check on my other patients."

"Thank you, Annya!"

The woman left the room. The man sat down beside Heinz's bed.

Heinz looked at him. He tried to move his tongue. It worked. He could speak, although slowly. "Schnitzel," he said with difficulty.

"Welcome back, Mr. Tremblay," the man said. "I don't think you are quite fit for dinner yet. And once you are, I bet you will be starting with soup in this establishment here."

"No—my—dog," Heinz managed to say.

"What about your dog?"

"You—have—him?"

"I'm sorry. I didn't see your dog anywhere."

Heinz started to breathe heavily. The pulse monitor beeped an alarm. His heart was racing. A nurse came running into the room. She looked at the FBI agent with disapproval. "Sir, if your presence upsets our patient here, then you'll have to leave."

The FBI agent raised both arms in defense. "I did not upset your patient. I'm here to protect him."

"Well, protect him without causing a heart attack, please."

"Yes, ma'am."

The nurse checked the monitor again. Heinz's heart rate slowly decreased back to normal values. She observed him for a few more minutes, then left.

"Please—find—my—dog," Heinz repeated.

The FBI agent pulled his cell phone. He showed him the photo of Nia, Ingrid, him, and Schnitzel from on his desk. "Is this your dog? A German shepherd?"

"Yes."

"Does he have a chip?"

"No."

"Well, that makes it a little more complicated. I assume he ran away. Your door was open. Is there any specific way we can recognize him?"

"Memory—drive—at—collar."

"So, he does have a chip after all?"

"USB—from—Nia."

"Your dog has a collar with an attached USB drive that contains information from Nia Johnes? The woman who was killed last night?"

"Yes."

"We will find your dog, Mr. Tremblay."

"Thank you."

The FBI agent stepped aside and talked with somebody on the phone. Then, he came back. "Why would you put a USB drive on your dog's collar?"

"Backup—from—laptop."

"Which laptop?"

"Nia's—laptop—my—office."

"I personally searched your office, but there was no laptop."

"Sure?"

"I'm certain that there was no laptop. Or did you hide it somewhere?"

"On—my—desk."

"Not anymore."

"What—about—Ingrid ?"

"Ingrid? Do you mean Ingrid Maulvi?"

"Yes"

"What about her?"

"She—was—there."

"Ingrid Maulvi was at your home today? We didn't see her."

The pulse monitor started beeping again.

"We will look for her as well, Mr. Tremblay. Does Ingrid know about the USB drive on the dog's collar?"

"No."

The nurse came back into the room. "With all due respect, it is time for you to leave, sir," she said to Terrel with a resolute tone.

Heinz looked at the FBI agent with a pleading gaze. "Please get some rest," Terrell said. "I will do everything I can to find your dog, Ingrid, and the laptop, okay?"

"Thank—you." Heinz tried to explain more, but the exhaustion overwhelmed him. He sank into a deep sleep.

- 21 -

LILI

Retaliation
Wednesday, May 25, 2033, 6:30 p.m.

Lili walked back to the research building. The sun had plunged behind the mountainside of the university promenade, outlining the leafy crowns of the majestic Redwood trees with a tapestry of intense gold, orange, and red colors. It was less busy than earlier today. Few people were walking up and down the hill, with some perhaps on their way home, and others taking photos of the valley below them. The drowning sun lulled the SUEC village into a glow of warm golden light.

It looked quiet and peaceful, but Lili surely knew that appearances could be deceiving. A cool breeze made her tighten her SUEC cardigan.

As she walked down the promenade, she let her thoughts wander. She felt relieved that she'd shared the results of the PCR tests with Dean Hill and agent Wright. They would take care of the next steps from here.

It had been a very long day, especially after her busy call night. Lili was tired. She would just fetch her laptop at her office and then head home.

When she approached the research building, she saw Dr. Robinson on the front porch, talking with somebody on his cell phone. He looked at her with a piercing gaze. Lili froze. *Telepathy does exist*, she thought. *He knows about the PCR tests.*

Dr. Robinson hung up the phone and stepped towards her with a friendly smile: "Oh, Lili, I'm glad to see you. Do you have a minute?"

Lili felt a cold shudder running down her spine. Again. This man just made her very uncomfortable. She had become weary of this combination of friendly voice and cruel gaze. Eye-mouth disconnection.

But what choice did she have?

"Of course, Dr. Robinson," she said politely.

They both walked into the building, through the lobby, up the stairs, through the lab, and into Dr. Robinson's office. It was like déjà vu. Lili had started to dread this view of the rainbow trees. And sitting down on the tacky golden leather seats. And talking with the vice dean.

He got right to the point. "Well, I'm afraid I have unexpected news: the majority of five evaluation letters for your promotion came back negative."

Lili's jaw dropped. She had expected some type of retaliation. But she had thought that the promotion process was following clear criteria, and could not be easily manipulated. "I have published more than 150 scientific publications," she managed to say. "That is almost twice as many as my colleague Matthew Holmes has published. And he was recently promoted."

Dr. Robinson looked at her with a wry smile. He was clearly enjoying the encounter. A predator eying his prey. "Well, as I explained earlier, we do not only consider such simple metrics as publications. We consider the entire person. You know, their social skills and professionalism."

"And what do the majority of five reviewers have to criticize about my professionalism?" Lili asked harshly.

"Lili, I understand that you are upset. But I'm only the messenger. I'm meeting with you after hours to inform you right away about an issue. So, be a little more polite, will you?"

"What is the issue?" Lili asked more loudly.

Two students in the lab next door looked up. Dr. Robinson waved at them with a broad smile, then turned back to her. "There are concerns that you have communication issues," he said calmly.

"Communication issues? Can you be a little more specific?"

Dr. Robinson walked over to his desk and opened a file on his computer. "Yes, of course, Lili. Let me read a summary to you."

He looked at the computer screen. "Our expert referees suggest that you need to do better to learn what to say out loud in front of others and what not to vocalize."

Lili did not believe her ears. Was it legal to treat her like this? "Is that so?" she said. "Does that not violate SUEC's freedom of speech? I thought that SUEC wants to encourage the expression of a wide range of viewpoints?"

Dr. Robinson did not respond, but continued to read from the screen. "Similarly, you need to be more sensitive to the effects of your actions on your colleagues and the reputation of the university."

"The effects of my actions? What actions?"

Dr. Robinson looked at her. "Lili, I want to help you here. I can confirm from my own observations that you sometimes act without considering the consequences."

"And what exactly do you think I should do better?"

"Focus on *your* research and *your* work. Don't get tangled up in other people's business. Remember, *any* faculty can be asked to provide feedback about you at any time. This feedback informs decisions about your appointment, your promotion, and your compensation. So, it is a good idea not to rub *anybody* the wrong way. It will backfire."

"You mean that people retaliate all the time here?"

"Don't offend me as well, Lili. I'm trying to help you. If your tenure application is denied, then your position here will not be extended. You'll lose your job at SUEC. But I will put a good word in for you. I will ask for an extension for another year so that you can sort out these issues. Then, we will reassess the situation next year, and hopefully, your evaluation will be positive then."

"I would like to receive the reasons for the denial of my promotion in writing," Lili said coldly.

"Certainly. You will receive an official notification letter," Dr. Robinson said smoothly. "In the meantime, make sure not to raise any new red flags."

Lili got up and walked out of the room.

Unfortunately, Jacub was not waiting for her at the door this time. Lili walked down the hallway and the spiraling staircase. One step. And another. And another.

She was shocked, disappointed, and disgusted. She was the only doctor in her family and had always felt privileged to be here. But deep inside, she felt that she did not belong. She longed for acceptance and approval, working twice as hard as her colleagues, literally around the clock.

She would prove herself. She thought that if not for her own person, her hard work would be appreciated. But that was an error. Her productivity was irrelevant. All that mattered here was politics.

Sparks of multicolored sunrays drizzled from the glass cupola into the foyer below her like a cloud of magic. The contrast of dazzling beauty and human cruelty was almost unbearable.

"Hello, Lili, I'm so glad you are still here!" Ying, one of her graduate students exclaimed. He was standing at the base of the stairs, looking up at her.

Not now, please. Lili felt so tired.

"I just noticed that the deadline for abstract submissions for the West Coast radiology symposium is today at midnight. I spent all afternoon putting a draft abstract together. Could you please have a look?"

Lili sighed. "Ying, you know our policy. You need to submit abstracts for my review at least forty-eight hours before the deadline. It is almost 7 PM right now. I'm afraid I won't have the time to look at it."

"I know it's my fault. I apologize. I somehow thought the deadline was two weeks from now—I'm pretty sure it was in June last year. It is really important for my career that I attend. I plan to apply for postdoctoral fellowships this year, and this will be a very important networking opportunity for me."

Should I teach him about concern for other people? She did not have the energy tonight. "You should have thought about it earlier, Ying. The submission deadlines are published months in advance. There's really no reason to make this an emergency."

"I know. I apologize. I spent extra time today to make the draft as perfect as possible. I promise it won't take much of your time. Can you please just have a quick look?"

Lili sighed. "Where is the abstract?"

Ying smiled. "You are the best PI in the world, Lili! I sent it to your email, and I put a hardcopy on your desk in your office."

Lili nodded. She walked back to her office and looked for her phone. It was not on her desk or in her pocket. She searched her entire office. Then she realized that she had been holding it in her hand the whole time. She was that exhausted. She called her husband Marc to tell him that she would be late, and that she might take a nap before coming home.

She did not want to end up in a car accident like Nia.

- 22 -

SCHNITZEL

The Abduction
Wednesday, May 25, 2033, 6:30 p.m.

Schnitzel woke up. It was completely dark, and he felt dizzy. Was it night already?

But he was not at Heinz's house. He was somewhere else. It smelled of used socks and underwear, mixed with the spice of dusty tree bark and damp moss. He was in some small confinement—a box, perhaps. He felt squeezed. He tried to stretch his limbs, but he could hardly move. The box was hard and narrow. And it was on the move. It rattled right and left, and he heard squeaking wheels below him. A suitcase?

There was a rapid change in odors that were passing by—people, other dogs, raccoon poop, flowers, a squirrel, pine trees, and the faint fragrance of a skunk in the distance. This wasn't a neighborhood he knew. The sheer quantity of new smells was overwhelming and nerve-wracking.

Schnitzel moved his nose around as much as he could. Scents informed his world. He was sure he hadn't been here before. And there was no smell of Heinz anywhere. Heinz was not here.

Instead, he picked up the sweet fragrance of the human who had tried to harm Heinz at their home. She smelled of a mixture of honey, eucalyptus tree, and disinfectant. Schnitzel had warned Heinz to stay away from her. But he did not listen. Why were humans sometimes so stupid? They had no sense for danger.

The suitcase stopped. Would she let him out now? His legs hurt. And his neck. It was too tight in here. And he could not breathe. Schnitzel heard the sound of a door being closed shut and noted the smell of freshly cooked human food—soup, fried potatoes, and grilled chicken. They were inside a building. He heard another door open and shut. A mechanical sound. An elevator. The woman did not say anything. She had to be alone. Still no hint of Heinz's familiar smell. Another door.

The suitcase was turned on its side and jammed Schnitzel's right ear against the hard plastic interior. He sent out a complaining bark. A blow hit the suitcase. Schnitzel took two 360-degree turns in his confinement. He started to bark frantically and pushed with his paws against the wall. He'd really had enough.

The smell of the human came closer. The suitcase opened. Schnitzel jumped out and bit the first thing that came into his way—a finger. The woman screamed. She had something in her hand. She leaped towards him. He felt a stinging pain in his backside. A syringe. He jumped at the woman. She leaped backwards, stumbled, and fell on her butt. Schnitzel went for the foot. She pulled it back, but he got a toe. She cursed.

His vision became blurry. He wanted to jump at her again, but his legs gave in. He collapsed.

And then it went dark again.

The haze in Schnitzel's brain slowly faded. He and Heinz were walking along the Russian River. Schnitzel loved the sound of the splashing water. It smelled of chlorine today. That was unusual. But Heinz was ruffling his head and assuring him that everything was okay.

They reached the sandy beach. Heinz took his shoes off, and they both waded into the water. Schnitzel's feet got wet. The chlorine odor became more intense. His nose got wet as well. He didn't like to dip his nose into the water. It was cold and smelled really unpleasant.

Something was not right. He opened his eyes. It was dark again. He lifted his head to get his nose out of the water, but he could only move a few centimeters above the waterline. His head hit a hard wall. A cave?

He remembered the suitcase. He was not at Russian River. Water *was* splashing beside him, and his feet were wet. In fact, his whole right side was wet. But this was not the Russian River. The stinging chlorine odor reminded him of something. His home. Upstairs. Heinz giving him a bath.

Schnitzel liked swimming in the Russian river, but he did not like being soaked in a bathtub. And this was not even Heinz's bathtub. He was not at home. He was in a bathtub somewhere else. No, he was in a suitcase in a bathtub. And the faucet was peeing. The water was coming into the suitcase.

Schnitzel started to panic. He tried to push and bite the suitcase open. But it did not move an inch. He started to howl as loud as he could. He needed help or he would drown!

- 23 -

CRISTINA

The Discovery
Wednesday, May 25, 2033, 6:30 p.m.

Cristina had a horrendous suspicion. To check it, she needed to get into Oliver's lab.

She slowly walked down the hallway. It was silent. The sound of talking people, clapping Erlenmeyer flasks, and walking feet had faded. Most researchers had left for the day.

Cristina peeked into Oliver's lab. He was still there, meeting with Lili in his office. The two were sitting on his ridiculous golden chairs, he talking and gesticulating, she glaring back. What was he harassing her about? Or was he making an advancement? Lili did not look like it.

And what did Cristina care? She and Oliver were done once and for all. Well, the sex had been amazing. But Oliver was a moral disaster. No values, no principles. No faith in anything. He liked to control people. Make them do things.

Lili looked really troubled. Poor thing. Hopefully, this conversation would not take too long.

Cristina walked back to her office and looked through the copies of the PCR tests again. She had studied them carefully. All of the samples appeared to have a common gene on the short arm of chromosome 3, at position 21. That was the CCR5 locus. Cristina wasn't an expert in IVF, but she knew this gene by heart. The C-C chemokine receptor type 5, also known as CCR5, was a protein on the surface of white blood cells that was involved in immune responses to infections. An inhibition of CCR5 had been discovered in people who were naturally resistant to the HIV virus. CCR5 also helped people fight off the effects of other infections.

In 2018, Chinese biophysicist He Jiankui had announced the birth of twin girls with edited CCR5 genes in an effort to make the children resistant to HIV infection. The problem was that changing the genome of an embryo could lead to unintended side effects, which would be inherited to generations to come. In 2020, experts from ten countries brought together by the US National Academy of Medicine, the US National Academy of Sciences, and the UK Royal Society had concluded that human embryos with edited genomes should not be used to create a pregnancy until it was established that precise genomic changes could be made reliably without introducing undesired changes. This milestone had not been reached yet by any genome-editing technology.

If Oliver or anyone in his team was editing CCR5 in human embryos and had implanted them, that would be against all current ethical conventions. And how had he done it? Nia and Ingrid were born before the CCR5 scandal. The technology hadn't been advanced enough at the time to edit embryos. According to the PCR results, Oliver was almost certainly their father.

Cristina tried to think how this could all be connected. Oliver had told her that his parents were from Europe. Approximately 10% of the European population carried the CCR5 mutation. What if he naturally had the gene for the CCR5 mutation and had just selected sperm with the desired gene combination? As a young man, he might have signed up as a sperm donor and just made sure he donated sperm with the CCR5 mutation. Later, once he had his IVF clinic, he could have selected sperm with the same mutation from other donors. Of course, some of the resulting embryos might not carry it, but he could similarly select the desired embryos with the CCR5 mutation and discard the ones that did not have it.

From there, he'd only need to sit back and observe what happened. It was both brilliant and scary.

Cristina heard footsteps on the hallway. She peeked around the corner and saw Lili walking down the stairs towards the lobby. She did not look back. A few minutes later, Oliver Robinson followed. He switched off the lights in the lab.

That should mean that everybody was gone.

To be sure, Cristina waited a few minutes longer. Then, she put on her white lab coat and slowly walked over to Oliver's lab. She stopped at one of the fume hoods and fetched two latex gloves from the glove box. She put them on. Then, she walked over to the storage room that contained the semen tanks, stainless steel containers that were used to store sperm for ART.

She looked around. How should she possibly identify the correct tank? All of them had a regular lid that could be easily opened, but one of them had a padlock on it. That had to be it! She walked over and inspected it. That shouldn't be too difficult. She took off her right shoe, which had a nice long and broad heel. When she grabbed it by the toe, the heel would make for a strong hammer. She inserted two fingers into the padlock's shackle loop and pulled on the shackle to create tension. Then, she tapped the side of the lock that contained the fixed end of the shackle with the shoe's heel with a few forceful strikes. The lock flung open.

Cristina opened the cover and took out the central plug. Vapor from liquid nitrogen came back at her. She knew that the temperature in the tank was around minus 300°F. She looked into the canister and saw a collection of straw-like tubes, the sperm containers. She reached into the container with a forceps, fetched five of the tubes, and put them in a thaw jar beside the canister. After a brief waiting period, she removed the thawed tubes and put them into the pocket of her white coat. She left the storage room and quickly walked through the lab towards the hallway.

When she walked out the door, she saw Oliver Robinson coming from the stairs towards the lab. He stopped and stared at her. "Hello, Cristina. What are you doing in my lab? Did you miss me?"

"Hello, Oliver. I thought I had heard Lili's voice here. I was looking for her. Did you see her, by any chance?"

He shook his head. "Cristina, you are a terrible liar. What is your nose doing in my business?"

"I was really only looking for Lili," Cristina responded with an innocent smile.

"Well, she's not here. But I'm available, if you're looking for a love interest. I always thought we were great together." He came closer.

If I googled horny, his picture would come up, Cristina thought. "I'm sorry, Oliver," she said with a charming smile. "I'm afraid our values do not align."

"Come on, Cristina. You're not that religious, after all. Or how does an affair square with the sixth commandment?"

"It doesn't. At the time, my husband had had an affair. Sleeping with you was my revenge."

"I find this a perfectly acceptable reason."

"I made a big mistake. And I paid for it." She waved around the lab. "This here violates the *Donum Vitae* and respect for human live."

He put his hand on her shoulder. "Cristina, I can assure you, I have the utmost respect for you."

Cristina stepped back. "I'm sorry I brought us into this impossible situation, Oliver. Whatever you think this was, it is over."

He looked at her with those enticing blue eyes. "You'll never find anyone like me."

"I sincerely hope so." Cristina slowly walked past him, her right hand wrapped around the tubes in her white coat. She turned around the corner, walked down the hallway, and went into her office. She felt Oliver's staring gaze on her back. She had to get out of here before he made another move. There seemed to be nobody else in the building, at least not on this floor.

She closed the door of her office, threw the tubes in her purse, grabbed her jacket, put it on, and opened the door again. He was still standing in the same spot, looking at her. "Cristina, tell me how I can change your mind. I'll do it. Anything you want," he said softly.

"Stop playing god. Close that IVF business of yours."

No response. *Of course.*

Cristina slowly walked down the stairs, through the lobby, and out of the building. She did not dare to look back. But she did not hear any footsteps behind her, either. So, hopefully, he was not following her.

Outside, she took a deep breath, her hand clutching her purse. The sun had started to set behind the Redwood hills, and a soft glowing twilight covered the silhouettes of the adjacent trees and the path in front of her. Few people were walking or biking up and down the small street that connected the research buildings with the SUEC village.

Was there somebody coming from the park towards her? A woman. She looked familiar. Was that Ingrid?

The woman looked at her, turned around and disappeared in the shadows of the park. Cristina slowly walked down the path to the street, then started running towards the village. Her knees felt wobbly.

That had been very close. If Oliver had come back a minute earlier, he would have found her in the storage room.

Soon enough, he would put two and two together.

- 24 -

OLIVER

The Plan
Wednesday, May 25, 2033, 6:30 p.m.

Oliver watched Cristina walking down the stairs, head high, carrying herself with alluring poise. Her long legs, her perfectly tailored silky dress, and her graceful movements were a stark contrast to the modern women nowadays in their flip-flops and shredded jeans. Beach clothes were for beaches, not work. Unless you worked at the beach, of course.

Cristina was the classiest woman he knew. She didn't need to show her naked skin to be seductive. Her beauty rivaled any movie star. Yeah, her stubborn head was a challenge sometimes, but Oliver liked her wit, her independence, and her confidence. She was like him: strong, smart, exceptional. Of course, she was not easy to get. He liked that about her as well. He was up for the challenge. His charm and persistence would get to her eventually. He knew she liked him.

He sent a hand-kiss in her direction, but she did not look back as she walked down the stairs to the atrium. He would try again tomorrow.

Oliver walked back to his office. Nathanael Zhang, the CEO of OrchidBio, was a man of his word. He had sent him a copy of his bid for licensing the patent. One billion dollars for an exclusive license and a ten-year research agreement. Oliver's family had always been well-off, but this would catapult him into the world of the super-rich. A mansion at the beach, a super yacht, a private jet, more fun—with Cristina at his side. And power. He would replace that stupid Dean and lead SUEC to new heights. More patents, more collaborations with industry, more wealth. And he would rule it all.

Oliver smiled as he sat down at his desk. Life would become really good. He opened the contract at his computer and read it carefully. Of course, his lawyers would have a look at the legal aspects of it, but he had to decide if he wanted to move forward with this transaction. Was it a good deal? Hard to say. Most patent-related transactions were strictly confidential and never became public. Known exceptionally lucrative acquisitions were the 6,000 Nortel portfolio for $4.5 billion and 925 AOL patents to Microsoft for $1.05 billion.

Of course, his commodity was particularly sensitive, as it involved an ethical gray area. However, the contract included substantial research investments that would spark new patents and new revenues. There were few people he could discuss this with, let alone starting an open licensing process. Nathanael was discreet and trustworthy. It was in his best interest to keep sensitive information under the lid. That would make the business all the more special.

Interested families would officially be enrolled in a research project at SUEC and unofficially receive a designer baby—a new must have for the rich and the wealthy. Rich people always wanted something new, and Oliver would deliver it to them. It was only a matter of time before the next pandemic struck. And their new generation of humans would be immune.

The contract looked great. Oliver felt satisfied and charged up at the same time. A sense of accomplishment and pleasurable anticipation. All the hard work had paid off. He had made it. A new world of wealth and power was waiting for him. He forwarded the contract to his trusted lawyer for the next steps.

Oliver hadn't noticed Ingrid coming into the lab. She suddenly stood in front of his desk. He closed the file. Another woman with shredded jeans, but he could forgive her. Firstly, she was young and beautiful. She could wear a trash bag and look gorgeous in it. Secondly, she was his daughter, and she loved him. The adoration in her eyes made him feel big and charismatic. Thirdly, this junk outfit would keep predators away, hopefully.

"I got the laptop," she said with pride in her voice, placing a MacBook Pro on his desk.

"Well done!" he said with an approving smile. He grabbed the laptop with both hands and placed it in his drawer. He would destroy it later tonight. *Get rid of the evidence ASAP.*

"But there was a complication: I got injured." Ingrid held her bloody finger in the air.

"What happened?" he said. "Let me have a look." He got up, walked around the desk, and inspected her finger.

"Heinz has a very aggressive dog. He attacked me."

Oliver walked to a cabinet behind the golden leather seats. He opened it and retrieved a small flask of disinfectant.

"Please sit down here." He pointed at the seat.

Ingrid shook her head. "It has to look authentic. When I was at the hospital this morning, the ER physician got very suspicious that I had cleaned the supposed gunshot wound with disinfectant. I do not want to make the same mistake again."

"It's an ugly wound," Oliver said. "And quite deep. It might get infected." He grabbed her hand and inspected it.

"Ouch. It really hurts," she said.

"And what is that?" Oliver pointed at a bloody toe in her sandal.

"Yeah, the dog bit my foot too. That one doesn't hurt as much as the finger."

"But it's quite swollen as well. You might need antibiotics."

Ingrid shook her head. "I get nauseated from those. I remember that from my previous infections. I was miserable."

"If this extends to the bone, it could get really bad very fast."

"Not for me."

"Well, don't be so sure about that. There are lots of things we don't understand yet. If it starts to produce pus, then you need to go to the hospital immediately."

"It won't. And as far as the dog is concerned, I doped him with ketamine and placed him in Cristina's apartment."

"In *Cristina*'s apartment? Why would you do that?"

"Because she and her friend Lili are snooping around. I do not want them to interfere with our project. I will disable her as you disabled Jacub."

"And how will a dog in her apartment accomplish that?"

"In a few minutes, I will go out on the street, call security, and tell them that I was drugged and abducted. I woke up in an unknown apartment and escaped. There was a frantic dog who bit me. The police will find the dog in Cristina's apartment and arrest her as a suspect."

Who would buy such a story? Oliver looked at Ingrid. She looked so innocent. And she was an excellent actress. It might work. But Cristina was smarter than her. She would surely talk herself out of this. He did not want her to get into any trouble. But if she did, he could come to her rescue. Oliver imagined himself as the knight who rescued the princess in distress. He liked it. "Well, I would be very interested to see if your scheme works," he said. "But either way, it will be a good distraction for the FBI agent. Perhaps you should call him."

"Yes, great idea. I got his number. He was hot."

That's daddy's girl, Oliver thought, smiling. "It would seem more natural if you just called 911," he said. "If the police find you, I am sure they will call Agent Wright as well. But keep SUEC out of this. Don't talk to any reporters. Ask the FBI agent to keep this confidential. We are about to license the patent and cannot have any negative publicity."

"Of course. I can tell him that I am concerned for my safety and that nobody should know that he found me."

"I will be impressed if they buy your story. But at the very least, you'll get proper dressing for your wounds."

"It doesn't matter if he believes me or not. If I report that I have been abducted, he must investigate the suspect. That will keep Cristina busy and prevent her from snooping around."

"I doubt that they'll arrest her. The FBI will need more evidence. And if Cristina can prove that *you* were lying, then *you* will be arrested."

"No worries. She won't. I love you, daddy," Ingrid said with a sweet voice. She hugged him lightly, then turned around and walked away.

Oliver looked after her. It was strange. He felt closer to Ingrid than to the two children he had raised. His daughter Lillian had no interest in science at all. Or any occupation, for that matter. She was currently trekking through Australia. His son Larry had just completed a clinical fellowship in obstetrics. He would become a fine medical doctor, but he did not have much interest in research either.

Ingrid was so excited about everything they did here at the ART lab. And she adored him. It would give him great satisfaction if she led the lab one day. Under his supervision, of course.

Then, he could fully focus on his new responsibilities as Dean of the university, all administrative aspects of his new business—and Cristina, of course.

- 25 -

CRISTINA

The Dog
Wednesday, May 25, 2033, 7:00 p.m.

Cristina arrived at her apartment building. Her husband's car was not there. It hadn't been for months. But nobody had noticed.

The semen samples fumed in her pocket. Some residual dry ice, perhaps. She was eager to bring the samples to a safe place. She walked up the stairs, taking two steps at a time. Her neighbor, Annya Segond, was standing in front of her door.

"Hello, Cristina," she greeted her. "I'm glad you're coming. I just wondered how I could get into your apartment. Since when do you have a dog?"

Cristina tried to catch her breath. "What are you talking about? I don't have a dog. I'm far too busy." She heard a howling sound coming from the inside of the apartment and looked at Annya, startled.

"Well, there is one in your apartment now. And he seems to be in distress."

Cristina fetched her keys and opened the door. Both women went in. Cristina looked around, shocked. What had happened here? The living room was in disarray. Two dining chairs were toppled over, the armchair was leaning against the window, shards of broken glass were scattered around the coffee table, and there were red stains on the carpet. Was that blood?

The sound of splashing water came from the right, along with a frantic howl. Annya ran into the bathroom, Cristina following her. There was a clawfoot bathtub in the back of the room. In it was an oversized, black hard-shell suitcase. The faucet was running. The water had reached the rim of the tub and was dripping on the black and white tile floor.

There was the howl again. It came from the suitcase.

"Oh, my God, there's a dog inside!" Cristina cried.

"Help me out here!" Annya shouted. She reached into the water and pulled the plug. Then she fetched the handle of the suitcase and pulled it out of the water. The howling intensified. Christina carefully placed her purse into the sink, then grabbed the other end of the suitcase. Water was pouring on the floor around them. They placed the suitcase on the floor.

"Step back!" Annya shouted. "I assume the hostage here will be very angry."

Cristina stepped back into the adjacent hallway and watched Annya through the open door. How could she be so calm? Cristina's heart was racing. She was soaked and scared.

Annya carefully released the latch of the suitcase. Then, she quickly jumped backwards. The suitcase flung open, and a German Shepherd jumped out of it. His tan-and-black coat was wet. He shook his body, covering his surroundings in a cloud of water drops, then looked up at Annya, walking stiffly towards her, his bushy tail up, hair standing on end, the square head boldly elevated, teeth bared, growling.

Cristina felt fear tightening her throat. She could hardly breathe. She retreated further down the hallway.

Annya did not move. She slowly turned side-on to the dog, lowered her body, made a hissing sound, and extended her right arm with an open palm. The dog stopped growling. Annya talked to him with a calm, soothing voice. "I'm sorry someone tried to drown you. That is horrible. You know it was not us."

The dog looked at Annya, his head tilted.

She came a little closer. "You must be exhausted. We are here to help you. You can trust us."

The dog slowly extended his long muzzle and sniffed her hand. Annya waited for a minute. Then, she extended her hand towards the dog and stroke his chest. He looked at her with dark, sad eyes. Annya moved her hand around and patted his head. He leaned into her.

"Wow, where did you learn that?" Cristina exclaimed from the hallway. "Are you a professional dog trainer?"

Annya smiled. "I adopted a pit bull from a shelter when I was a young woman. We went to dog school together. His name was Jimmy. It was a great learning experience for both of us."

"But he doesn't live here with you?" Cristina said.

"Well, that was a long time ago. He died."

"I'm sorry."

"Let's focus on the dog here. What is he doing in your apartment?"

"I have no idea. I've never seen him before." Cristina looked at the dog. Who had put him into her apartment? And why?

Annya took photos of the bathroom and the dog with her iPhone. Then, she walked past Cristina into the living room and took additional photos there. Cristina fetched her purse and followed her. "Don't touch anything," Annya said. "This is a crime scene. The police might be able to get some fingerprints here. Call security."

Cristina nodded, then called the number of the SUEC security team. Two minutes later, two security guards arrived. They interviewed the two women and then started investigating the scene.

"Would you like to wait in my apartment next door?" Annya asked. "I can make us a tea and sandwich. I presume you haven't eaten anything yet?"

"No, I haven't. A tea would be lovely."

The two women went into Annya's apartment next door. The dog followed them. They entered the small modern kitchen, which featured a bright parquet floor, a big stainless-steel oven, dishwasher and refrigerator, and shiny birch cupboards with stainless steel handrails that matched the appliances. A few anemic plants in hand-painted porcelain pots were lined up along the window shelf. Annya took a beautifully crafted porcelain teapot from the cupboard and turned to the stove to prepare the tea.

"This is beautiful!" Cristina exclaimed.

Annya smiled. "It is a Zavarnik, a traditional Russian teapot. It will take just a minute."

Cristina looked around. The back of the room led to a French door with a small balcony. "Do you mind if I open the doors?" she asked.

"Sure, go ahead."

Cristina opened the doors. A fresh breeze entered the room. It was a beautiful summer evening. "Oh, you have stairs leading down to the garden?" she noted.

Annya nodded. "I am the only one who has these. I had them custom-made when I moved in. I like to have multiple options when it comes to entering or leaving my home. Plus, it gives me direct access to the garden."

The dog joined Cristina, exploring the area. He slowly walked onto the balcony, then down the steep stairs. "Do you think it is okay for him to go down there?" she asked.

Annya nodded. "The garden is fenced; I think it's fine. He probably needs to do his business."

Cristina watched the dog as he climbed down the stairs. When he had reached the ground, she turned around and saw Annya with a tray in her hands. She was carrying a steaming teapot, two sandwiches, a small plate with sliced lemon, and a sugar bowl. "Wow, that was fast," Cristina said.

"I am not a particularly good cook, but I'm very time-efficient. I have to be," Annya responded with a smile.

They went into the sparsely furnished living room that featured an electric fireplace, an emerald-green Chesterfield sofa with two side tables, and a lacquered rosewood Art Deco dining table with four vintage dining chairs. The women sat down at the table. Cristina only realized now how hungry she was. They both ate calmly for a while. The tea was sweet and strong. Revitalizing.

Cristina reached for her purse. "Annya, I have a special request."

Annya looked at the purse. "What is that?"

"SUEC hospital has a very sophisticated genomics lab, right?"

"Yes, it does. Why are you asking?"

"Well, could you request an analysis of a few samples for me?"

"What samples?"

Cristina opened her purse so that Annya could see the test tubes inside. "I have a suspicion. I know it sounds crazy, but please hear me out. We found PCR tests that show that Ingrid and Nia and another person with first name Heinz are half-siblings. In addition, we found that Oliver Robinson is most likely their father."

Annya looked at her with wide eyes. "Dr. Robinson is Ingrid *and* Nia's father? That can't be true. Does Terrel know about that rumor?"

"Yes, I gave him the tests so that he can double check."

"Okay. You're in the best hands." Annya refilled her teacup.

"Well, I found something else: Ingrid, Nia, Heinz, and Oliver all have a mutation of the CCR5 gene—a gene that makes people resistant to infections. Oliver is the world expert in assisted reproduction techniques. I'm wondering if he is selecting sperm, eggs, or embryos with this mutation to create infection-resistant babies. Sperm would be technically the most straightforward, I think."

"That's quite a fantastic idea."

"I know. Perhaps my imagination went too far, but usually, my sixth sense works very well. So, today I had a look in Oliver's lab. And guess what? I found a semen tank with a lock on it. That is quite unusual. I borrowed a few specimens from that tank."

"You stole sperm samples?"

"Well, there were multiple samples per donor; it won't be such a big loss."

"Says the thief who is an adamant opponent of assisted reproduction. You know that you can get into big trouble for that? I suggest you return the samples ASAP."

"Yeah, you are right. Perhaps I will get in trouble. But one of my students has been murdered, and it turns out that she is the daughter of the colleague next door. She was conceived by IVF, and she studies IVF. This has to have something to do with her death. I'm just trying to understand what is going on here. Could you take the samples to the genetics lab and analyze them?"

Annya looked at her for a while. Then she nodded. "Perhaps you are on to something. I know the chief technician in the lab. I will talk with him."

"Thank you!" Cristina flipped the purse over the cresting rail of Annya's chair. "Please keep this confidential for now. Perhaps I'm totally wrong. I do not want to distribute any false accusations. Oliver is egotistic and power-hungry, but he was always kind to me, even if I offended and insulted him."

"Yes, I agree. Let's get the facts straight first. It's much more likely that we'll find nothing than that your theory will prove to be true."

Cristina nodded. There was a brief moment of silence.

"Do you want to call your husband and warn him that he'll find the security team in your living room when he gets home? He seems to be working very long hours lately."

"Well, he moved out. We split about a year ago."

"Oh?"

"I didn't want Oliver to know. Or anybody else, for that matter. I'm not interested in a new relationship at the moment."

"I understand."

"You are single as well?"

Annya nodded. "Yeah, I made bad choices when I was young. I was married to a Russian spy and serial killer. For several years, I had no idea that he lived a double life. When I found out and tried to get away, I nearly got killed." She lifted her bangs and pointed to a big scar on her forehead.

"Wow, that's terrible. Are there no happy relationships anymore? I mean, couples who live ordinary lives, who love each other, and who are together for the long run. Until death takes them apart."

"Well, I guess relationships have become more nuanced in our modern times. Many people live together for a while and then continue on different paths. But some couples seem to be happy together for a very long time. Terrel Wright is very fond of his wife Imani and his little son Niles. Lili has been happily married to her husband Mark for more than twenty years. And Robert Hill is happily married to his husband Atharv, and they are about to adopt a baby girl."

Cristina sighed. "Yeah, I guess we're just the unlucky ones."

Annya cleaned her mouth with a napkin. "First, I think I'm happy right now. Second, I haven't given up on romantic relationships. I'm just not forcing it. If the right person comes along, great. If not, I'm perfectly content with myself."

Cristina stirred sugar in her teacup. "I am just wondering if I'll lose my time window to have children. Are you afraid that you might die alone?"

"Who says that people with kids would *not* die alone? Once your children are grown up, they will likely live elsewhere or be occupied with their own lives. There's no guarantee that they'll care for you when you're old. I would say a circle of close friends is a pretty good alternative."

Cristina nodded. "I just wished that life would be less painful."

Annya patted her shoulder. "This will pass. One day, you'll share your story about your struggles, and it will help someone else."

The balcony door in the kitchen rattled in the wind. Annya got up and walked over. Cristina followed her, carrying the tray with the empty plates. They had to get the dog in.

Annya stepped on the balcony and whistled. No response. It was getting dark outside. The solar torches on the small yard had started to emit a flickering light. The perfectly groomed artificial lawn in the middle was empty. There was no dog anywhere.

"I don't understand," Cristina said. "He cannot run away; the fence is at least six feet tall."

Annya looked around. "Well, there's no space to hide down there."

They walked down the stairs and along the perimeter of the fence, looking behind the palm trees and checking every bush. There was no hole in the fence, but there was no dog either. He was gone.

The doorbell rang. Annya walked back up to open it. Cristina followed. There were two police officers at the door. One of them asked, "Is Mrs. Walker-Díaz here?"

Not this again. "Do you mean Dr. Walker-Díaz?" Annya asked politely.

"Yes, the woman who owns the apartment next door."

"I'm here." Cristina stepped forward.

"Ma'am, we have to ask you to come with us to the police office. We have a few questions for you."

Cristina looked at Annya. "Can you ask her here?" Annya asked.

"I'm afraid an injured woman has been found on the street who claims that she was kidnapped by Mrs. Walker-Díaz. We found her fingerprints in your apartment."

"Kidnapped by *me*?" Cristina exclaimed. "Dr. Segond here can attest that I just came home about an hour ago. We rescued a dog in my apartment. If I had put him there, why would we rescue him? Besides, I was in the SUEC research building all day long and have numerous witnesses who can confirm this."

"Sorry ma'am. We're just doing our job."

"This is ridiculous! How should these hands kidnap anyone?" Cristina held up her hands to show her long, perfectly manicured nails.

"It's just a routine interview at this time," the officer said. "Please come with me. I really hope that I don't have to apply any force here."

Annya patted Cristina's hand. "It'll be okay. They cannot arrest you without evidence. Just comply and provide them with any information that you know. Perhaps you can help finding the kidnapper. And who knows? Perhaps this is the same person or same group that killed Nia."

Cristina nodded. "I guess I don't have a choice, do I?"

"Thank you, ma'am," the officer responded. "Hopefully, it won't take too long."

Cristina fetched her jacket and followed the two officers.

Annya watched her disappear down the hallway. Then, she went back into the living room, grabbed the purse that Cristina had given her, and left the apartment. She would get the samples analyzed now.

- 26 -

SCHNITZEL

The Escape
Wednesday, May 25, 2033, 7:15 p.m.

Schnitzel explored the artificial grass in the backyard of the apartment building. There were several coagulates of intensely smelling dog urine, that had built up between the bottom of the grass carpet and the weed barrier beneath it. Disgusting.

He looked up to the apartment building. The entrance to the kitchen was illuminated, and he heard the two women talking inside. He liked them, especially the one who smelled like magnolia, blood, and a hint of disinfectant. She had rescued him. He would not forget that. The other one exuded a little too intense fragrance for his muzzle, a mixture of jasmine, vanilla musk, and roses, coupled with the smell of vinyl gloves. Her sad mood was hard to bear, and her purse was outright scary. It smelled of dead men and Ingrid. It reminded him of being crammed in the suitcase.

He was still shaken by the recent events and was glad to be in the open now. Schnitzel trotted around the small yard. More dog urine. This was clearly somebody else's pitiful territory. Where was Heinz? He missed him so much. And Nia.

He heard a familiar sound behind the fence. Two people were talking. "Nia…Nia…Nia."

That needed to be investigated. Schnitzel stood still and held his pointed ears as high as possible. There it was again. "Nia…Nia…Nia."

He did not recognize the voices, but these humans clearly knew Nia. If they knew her, perhaps they knew Heinz as well. He had to get to them.

He looked at the fence. It wasn't that tall. He took a few steps back. Then he raced towards the fence and jumped. He tried to get traction with his feet on the top of the fence and pull himself up, but his front paws slipped off and he fell back. He stepped back again. To his right, there was a large bin leaning against the fence. That would help. He sprinted towards it, jumped on the bin, up the fence, hooked over the top of the fence, hauled himself over it, and jumped down the other side.

He had done it! He felt a proud sense of victory.

Schnitzel found himself on a lawn beside a small street lined with perfectly manicured palm trees and limestone buildings. Few humans were walking up and down the sparsely lit sidewalk, and there were no dogs, who would have easily spotted him. Schnitzel stayed in the shadows of the fence and listened. Where were the humans? He did not hear their voices anymore.

He raised his muzzle into the air. To his right was the smell of perfume—too strong for his nose—and two young women whispering something to each other. To his left, he detected the fragrance of the food that Nia had sometimes brought to Heinz's place: Caribbean roti, stewed meat, and vegetables folded tightly in a round flatbread. Delicious. Nia had often shared a bite with Schnitzel, despite Heinz's half-hearted protest. He had particularly liked the one with the meat. Saliva filled his mouth. Left it was.

Schnitzel followed the lead. He suppressed the urge to chase a daring squirrel that crossed his path. The roti scent came closer. There was a human couple in front of him, a man and a woman, walking hand in hand. The man was muttering something. The woman was giving out constant sniffles and high-pitched sighs, dropping a steady stream of salty tears on the hot pavement.

Schnitzel felt overwhelmed by her profound sadness. *What desolate, melancholic place is this,* he thought. *Everyone I met is miserable.*

Schnitzel slowed down and followed the couple patiently. They took a left turn into a small path that led into the Redwood forest. The trees along the path had blue string lights on them. The adjacent bushes were covered in a slight mist. Schnitzel's fur got damp, and the air around him got a few degrees colder. It smelled good of dusky bark, deer, pinecones, and moss. Schnitzel fetched a Redwood branch on the forest floor and took it along.

They'd walked along the path for about ten minutes when a white building with a bell tower appeared at the end—a chapel. Two twisting Solomonic columns with carved sculpted vines flanked the ornate entrance. The woman said something to the man, then opened the rustic oak door and disappeared inside.

The man walked towards a bench to the left of the building. As he turned around to take a seat, he noticed Schnitzel. The man froze for a moment, observing the large dog.

Schnitzel tried to make a friendly impression. He sat down in front of the man, looked at him with his soft dark eyes, and placed the redwood branch at his feet.

"Where did you come from?" the man grunted. He looked around. "Did you get lost? Where is your human?"

He searched in his pocket, produced a chocolate-chip cookie, and offered it to him. Schnitzel slowly came closer, sniffed at the cookie, and gratefully accepted it. He had forgotten how hungry he was.

"Good boy. You are a real beauty!" The man produced another cookie and patted Schnitzel's head as he was chewing. He was a nice man, and generous. Schnitzel liked him a lot.

Suddenly, they heard a growling sound behind them. The man's eyes widened. Schnitzel turned around and saw a coyote standing under the trees, baring his teeth, gauging the man's and Schnitzel's ability to respond. Schnitzel was unimpressed. The snarling dog was a third his size, and Schnitzel would gladly consume him for dinner, but the old man on the bench was scared. Schnitzel smelled his cold sweat. And likely so did the coyote. That was no good.

Schnitzel hunkered down to look small. The coyote came closer. Schnitzel jumped up, ready to engage and teach this chap a lesson. But to his surprise, the old man jumped up as well and threw a big stone at the coyote. Not bad. The coyote howled and retreated backwards. The man threw a few more pinecones at him, as well as the branch that Schnitzel had brought him.

Schnitzel was impressed. He had found a hero! He wanted to add his part and charge after the coyote, but the man grabbed him by his collar and held him back. The coyote turned around and disappeared in the woods.

"We don't want to get injured," the man murmured as he stroked Schnitzel's back. Schnitzel leaned against the man. He sat back down on the bench, and Schnitzel put his big head on his knees. The man scratched him behind his ears. He liked that. Now, the man examined his collar.

The door of the church opened, and the woman came back. She sat down beside the man. "This was good," she said. "I feel as if I can talk with her from the church bench. I miss her so much."

"I know. I miss her too."

"You found a new friend here?" She pointed at Schnitzel.

Schnitzel focused his full attention on her, nuzzling her hand and wagging his tail. She scratched his head and sighed. "Nia would have liked you. She was always so good with dogs."

Schnitzel confirmed with a brief bark.

The women looked at the man. "He reminds me of Polly, Nia's first dog. She was crazy about him."

The man looked at her, tears welling up in his eyes. "Every time I see a German Shepherd, I think of her."

The woman nodded. "I know what you mean. I remember how she ran through the woods with Polly, throwing and fetching sticks, laughing. I remember how she tended to run her fingers across his fur, and how he jumped up and licked her all over her face."

"And the dog following her everywhere, just like this chap here."

"Did this dog get lost?" the women asked.

"It appears so. He has a memory stick on his collar." The man pulled gently on Schnitzel's collar, parted his thick fur, and showed the memory stick to the woman.

"That's unusual," she said.

"Well, we are at SUEC. Perhaps dogs do not wear simple GPS chips anymore. Perhaps there is some information about him on this memory stick—the name or phone number of his owners. We can check and then call them."

"For that, he needs to come with us. Do you have a leash?"

"No, but I think he will come with us regardless. He chose us, not the other way around."

"Hm, let's try." The woman got up from the bench. The man followed her. So did Schnitzel.

"See, I told you so."

The woman smiled. Schnitzel stayed close to her. Perhaps he could lift her mood.

The three walked back to the village.

- 27 -

TERREL

The Plan
Wednesday, May 25, 2033, 7:30 p.m.

Terrel arrived on the rooftop of the Phillip Burton Federal Building at Golden Gate Avenue in downtown San Francisco in an eVTOL aircraft. The massive twenty-one-floor building occupied an entire city block near San Francisco's Civic Center, and the rooftop provided ample space for multiple simultaneously departing and landing aircrafts. The evening fog rolled in pale wisps and dark waves over the rooftop, embracing Terrel with teeth-shattering damp coldness.

He got out of the eVTOL and fought his way against the icy wind to the building entrance. He took the elevator to the thirteenth floor, where the Federal Bureau of Investigation was located. He had received important updates from the forensic lab, which he wanted to share with Jacub Bezdomny. The SUEC building manager would be pleased. The FBI team had done an excellent job.

Jacub was already waiting for him in the main conference room, with FBI agent Lamong Setang at his side. Terrel nodded briefly at Lamong as he walked in. He was one of his best men. Jacub was sitting at the rectangular laminate conference table, his shirt torn and dirty, his hair in disarray, arms folded in front of his chest. Terrel moved two untouched water bottles to the side and took a seat across from him. Jacub looked at him with an angry gaze. Or was it fear? Probably a bit of both. Time to release the pressure.

"Hello, Mr. Bezdomny. I have good news for you," Terrel said calmly. "You have been cleared, and you can go home shortly."

Jacub led out a sigh of relief. "I told you I was innocent! How have I been cleared?"

"The fingerprints on the gun and your current fingerprints are different. You have a deep cut on your index finger. Footage from the security video of the SUEC research building showed that you injured your finger while cutting the rose bushes in front of the research building on Monday, one day before Nia was shot. Your fingerprints on the gun don't show this cut. Therefore, they must be from any time before Monday. They have been planted on the gun."

"That's what I said the whole time!" Jacub exclaimed.

"I know. But we had to find evidence first to exonerate you."

"This was a hell of a day. I really thought I would end up in jail or worse. Who planted a gun in my office?"

"I don't know that yet, but our team here will find out. Do you have any enemies, Mr. Bezdomny?"

"You mean someone who wants to frame me for murder? I didn't think so until today. I'm just a building manager. What threat could I be to anyone? I'm far too unimportant."

"You live in your office in the research building?"

Jacub looked at the FBI agent with raised eyebrows. "How did you find that out?"

"Mr. Bezdomny, you're talking with the FBI."

Jacub turned his gaze to the white laminate tabletop in front of him. "Well, it is the Bay Area, you know; housing is expensive. My office has everything I need."

"But you get a pretty generous compensation at SUEC."

"Yeah, but if I rented an apartment, most of it would be wasted. If I live in my office for a few years, I'll save a lot of money, and can buy an apartment, either here or in Poland, where I come from. In fact, in Poland, I could buy a big house."

"Did the SUEC administration ever comment on your personal arrangement?"

"I'm not sure if anybody has noticed. As I said, I'm far too unimportant. If they noticed, they probably didn't mind. I provide 24/7 supervision of the research building."

"And with that, you know your tenants much better than the average manager?"

Jacub smiled faintly. "I guess so."

"You would see who stays late?"

"Yeah, I usually walk through the building and make sure everyone is gone before I get a beer and turn on the TV in my office. I want to keep a low profile, you know. If somebody is working late, then I go to the gym or take a walk through the park, then check again before I settle for the night."

"Did anybody stay late on May 24, the night Nia was killed?"

"Yes, both Cristina Walker-Díaz and Ingrid Maulvi stayed late that night. Cristina worked on her computer in the lab. She asked me to bring her a pizza and a Coke from that store next door. She left around 8:30 PM. I walked by Dr. Robinson's lab and saw that Ingrid was working late as well."

"Did she order something too?"

"No, she never orders anything. Cristina is always up for a chat, but Ingrid hardly talks to me at all."

"Do you know how long Ingrid stayed in the lab that night?"

"Not exactly. I went to the diner down the street for dinner. When I came back around 9 PM or so, she was gone. But the lights were still on in the lab, and her jacket was hanging over her chair. That was annoying. I took a walk through the park. When I checked again around 10 PM, the lights were out, and she and her jacket were gone."

"Thanks, that might be helpful."

"Do you think Ingrid shot Nia?"

"I'm still collecting evidence. What do you think?"

"Well, Ingrid and Nia had some argument in the foyer here a few days ago—yelling at each other like their lab directors. These postdocs are like kids, you know. I thought that Cristina and Oliver were bad role models. They argue with each other all the time, so their team members fight as well. Ingrid and Nia did not like each other, but I cannot imagine they would shoot each other."

Terrel nodded. "Mr. Bezdomny, I would like to request your assistance."

"My assistance? Locking me up in chains and accusing me of murder is not the best foundation for asking for a favor."

"Well, let's call it a transaction, then. I won't tell anybody about your housing arrangement, and you will help me out here."

Jacub stared at Terrel. "You are blackmailing me?

"Well, I would rather call it an agreement."

Jacub looked at him for a while. "What do you want me to do?"

"It's very simple: I want to place a microphone on your blazer. We'll hide it behind an SUEC lapel button."

"And what do you want me to record?"

"There are many interactions in that research building that we do not understand yet. They could be a clue about the cause for all this violence. You have a natural talent for monitoring what is going on. You're always where the action is. Just be your usual self. We'll take care of the rest."

"And you won't tell anybody that I live in my office?"

"I don't think that's FBI business, is it?"

Jacub nodded. "Thanks. I'll help you find the killer."

"Excellent!" Terrel pointed to the FBI agent beside Jacub. "My colleague Lamong here will get you outfitted and drive you back to the university. Thanks for your service!"

Terrel left the conference room. That had gone very well. He now had ears on the inside, and he could locate Jacub at all times through the GPS chip in the lapel button.

Terrel checked his iPhone. It had buzzed multiple times during their conversation. He read: *Break-in at Cristina Walker-Díaz's apartment. Nobody injured. German shepherd rescued.*

This was too much of a coincidence. It had to be Heinz's dog. The dog with a memory stick glued to his collar. Terrel texted back, *Secure the dog. Important evidence.*

There was another text message from the head of the SUEC security team: *Ingrid Maulvi found on a road north of SUEC. She was kidnapped and escaped. Major injuries. Checked in to SUEC hospital.*

Terrel texted back, *OMW.*

- 28 -

OLIVER

Interventions
Tuesday, May 25, 2032, 8 p.m.

The melodic voice of Oliver Robinson's digital assistant reminded him of the time: 8 PM. That meant time to go home.

He shut down his computer and distributed the pieces of Nia's shredded laptop to three different trash cans in the lab. Not his office, of course. The hard drive was destroyed beyond retrieval, but he wanted to make sure no trace led to him. The cleaning lady would discard them tonight.

Oliver walked back to his office, took a comb and mirror out of his desk drawer, and straightened his hair. It had been a long day, but he looked good. He felt energized by the prospect of the patent deal. He would pick up a bottle of champagne on the way home and surprise his wife, Sylvia.

They had seen better times. They were estranged, pretty much living parallel lives by now. She focused on the children, he on the job. When he came into the bedroom at night, she was sleeping. When he got up in the morning, she was sleeping. The fire of their early relationship had long-since drowned in their daily routine.

Oliver had often planned to discuss the matter with her and file for divorce. But who would move out? Oliver was so busy with his job. He had no time for this. Sylvia was a wonderful mother to his two children, and she was an excellent cook. It wasn't a good time right now. Maybe later.

Today, they would celebrate!

Someone knocked at his office door. Oliver looked up and saw Andrew, one of the SUEC security guards, behind the glass door. "Hello Dr. Robinson, do you have a minute?"

"Of course, Andrew! What's the matter?"

"I made an important observation, and I think it might be related to the shooting of the student in this building."

Oliver leaned back in his chair. "And what did you discover?"

"Well, you might remember that SUEC supports a biannual dibling party, where people who were conceived through the same sperm or egg donor can get to know each other. The latest dibling party was in January in the assembly hall at SUEC. Yesterday, Agent Wright asked me to review the security videos of the last dibling party and check if I found anything unusual. Well, I found something." He paused and produced a memory stick from his pocket.

"What is this?" Oliver asked.

"Please see for yourself." The guard handed him the memory stick. Oliver restarted the computer and pulled up the drive, which contained a video clip. Oliver double-clicked the file, and the video started. It showed a colorfully decorated room with balloons and flower garlands. Multiple round tables with white table linens and beautiful flower centerpieces were scattered throughout the room. Chatting young people were sitting at the tables. Androids were delivering plates with food. Several of the young people were taking photos.

"Look at this." The guard pointed at a table at the far-right end of the room. *Was Ingrid sitting there?* Oliver adjusted his glasses. *Yes, it's her!* She was talking with an attractive-looking young Asian man. They both cheered their wine glasses. An android approached with food plates, and the young man turned away from Ingrid to grab them. She quickly reached into her pocket, produced a tiny flask, and dropped some fluid into his wine glass. When the man turned back towards her, the flask had disappeared in her pocket.

"Hm, that is interesting," Oliver said, chuckling. "I thought guys spiked women's drinks, not the other way around."

The guard's cheeks flushed. "Well, I investigated this further. Both the man and Ingrid departed from the party separately and at different times. They both live on campus, and I did not notice any inappropriate advances, but I identified the man with face-recognition software and discovered that he went to the SUEC emergency room the next day. There, he was diagnosed with infectious enteritis. I actually got a copy of his CT scan." The guard pointed to another file on the memory stick.

Oliver opened it. It showed a CT scan of the abdomen with a brief note: *Multiple thickened and edematous small bowel loops in the upper and mid abdomen. Edematous swelling of the submucosa, the outer lining of the bowel wall, and hyperemic, contrast enhancing mucosa, the inner lining of the bowel wall. These findings are highly suggestive of an infectious enteritis.*

Oliver turned to the security guard. "Thank you for bringing this to my attention, Andrew! I'm glad you came to me first. Of course, we don't want to draw any premature conclusions here. Who knows what Ingrid put into his drink? It seems unlikely that it has to do with his hospital visit, but I will certainly investigate this carefully."

"And you will hand it over to the FBI?"

"Yes, of course. Consider it taken care of!"

"Thank you, Dr. Robinson."

"For now, keep this confidential, will you? We don't want to create any gossip. SUEC's reputation has already taken a hit with the news about Nia Johnes's death. We do not want to saw off the branch on which we are sitting."

"Of course not." The guard bowed slightly.

Someone else cleared his throat. Oliver looked around and saw Jacub standing in the door with a handful of envelopes. *Why is this guy not locked up? And how long has he been standing there?*

"Hello, Dr. Robinson. I brought your mail," he said cheerfully.

"At 8:15 p.m.?" Oliver asked sharply.

"I'm very sorry for the delay; I was indisposed earlier today," Jacub said.

"Thank you," Oliver said, snatching the envelopes from Jacub's hands. "I have sensitive business to attend to. Would you please give me some privacy?"

"Of course," Jacub said. "I wish you a wonderful evening!"

The security guard looked from Oliver to Jacub, then bowed again, turned around, and walked away. Jacub followed him.

Oliver watched both men traverse the lab, turn around the corner, and disappear down the hallway. He was furious. Who had released this nosy building manager? He picked up the phone and called the cell phone number of Angus Weber, FBI director.

"Hello, Angus, this is Oliver Stuart Robinson from SUEC. How are you doing?"

"Busy, as usual. I heard about the incident with the student. I hope this doesn't evolve into something bigger. How can I help?"

"Well, I wanted to consult you on a delicate matter. I know you want to give Agent Wright a chance leading the investigations here. He is young and ambitious, and I like him a great deal, but I am afraid this project is too big for him."

"Terrel Wright is my best man. If the shooter is still out there, he will find him."

"I am afraid I cannot share your enthusiasm. Yesterday, an SUEC student was shot. Today, my lab manager Ingrid Maulvi was assaulted. Agent Wright seems completely clueless about what is going on. I was informed by SUEC personnel that an unidentified man is walking around campus with a gun. More shockingly, this person had the audacity to record Agent Wright's conversations with a cell phone. It seems that criminals are surveying Agent Wright, not the other way around."

"Thanks for bringing this to my attention. I will look into it."

"I need more than words, Angus. I am concerned for my own safety and that of the SUEC community. Earlier today, a gun was found in the office of our building manager. Agent Wright arrested him, but just a minute ago, this man was walking into my office. Apparently, he was released. Can you tell me why? I am concerned about the safety of everyone in this building."

"Sorry, I'm not appraised of every detail of the investigation."

"You should be. SUEC is the crown jewel of our country, a major drive to innovation and economic power. If news about crimes at SUEC spreads, we could lose donor support and billions in investments. This incident severely damages our reputation and that of the FBI. It will look like criminals are dancing on your nose. You need to solve this now!"

"I hear you. I will personally debrief Agent Wright and inform you as soon as we have any news."

"What about the man with the gun in the building here?"

"I will check on that as well. As I said, Agent Wright is my best man. He would not release the man if he had any evidence that he could be a danger to others."

"Well, he had a gun in his office."

"I will find out what happened and get back to you."

"I look forward to hearing from you very soon." Oliver hung up.

Mission accomplished! He now had a hot wire to the FBI investigation and could warn Ingrid if needed.

Oliver grabbed his jacket. Finally, time to go home. The patent deal was as good as sealed. He *would* open a bottle of champagne tonight. He only wished he could drink it with Cristina. One move at a time. She would come around eventually.

Oliver left the office and walked through the lab. Someone had left the door open to the storage room. He grunted with disapproval. He had grabbed the handle to close the door shut when his gaze fell on something shiny on the ground. He stepped into the storage room to pick it up. *What the hell?* A broken padlock!

He walked to the semen tank in the back of the room. Someone had broken into it. Oliver's thoughts raced. Who had done this? He hadn't noticed the open door when he walked past here less than an hour ago.

It had to be the building manager. He knew too much. If the building manager told anyone about the sperm samples, Oliver's entire enterprise was in jeopardy. This man had gone too far. Oliver couldn't tolerate this.

He went down the stairs and to Jacub's office. Jacub was sitting on his couch, eating a slice of pizza and watching a soccer game on his laptop. He looked at Oliver in surprise. "Hello, Dr. Robinson, can I do something for you?"

"Oh, Jacub, you are still here?"

"Yeah, I wanted to make sure everyone in the building is safe. I will leave after the last tenant has left."

"That is very noble of you."

"No problem. These are difficult times for all of us."

"Since you're still here, I was wondering if you can help me with a problem."

Jacub's eyes were on the computer screen. The midfielder had acquired the ball and was running towards the goal. "Can it wait until tomorrow?" he asked politely.

"Of course—whenever you get a chance," Oliver responded. "I'm having issues with the 7G network. The internet connection in my office is very slow. The last time that happened, there was something wrong with the antenna on the roof."

"My computer here works just fine."

"Well, that doesn't help me, does it?"

"Sure, I'll have a look."

"I have a phone conference early tomorrow morning. It would be great if it was working again by then."

"Of course. I'll fix it."

"Thank you!" Oliver turned around and walked towards the foyer. Instead of walking towards the exit, he went back up the stairs. At the top of the stairwell was a small door that led onto the roof. It was dark outside. Faint lights from the streetlamps illuminated the small fenced balustrade that led to the cupola. The five-foot-tall antenna was secured to the east base of the shiny glass dome.

Oliver cowered behind a large pillar. He did not have to wait long.

About fifteen minutes later, Jacub stepped onto the balustrade. He walked toward the antenna and inspected it with a flashlight. He exhaled sharply. Everything was in proper order. He turned around, his back facing Oliver.

Oliver leaped forwards and pushed Jacub forward as hard as he could. Jacub cried out and flew headfirst over the balustrade, his hands waving wildly through the air as if he were trying to hold onto something. But there was nothing.

Oliver observed with fascination how Jacub's body first flew upwards and then transitioned to a hyperbolic downward trajectory. Jacub led out an animalistic cry. There was a dull sound as his body hit the paved path in front of the building.

Then, there was silence.

Oliver dusted off his trousers, then went down the stairs and out of the building towards the street. He saw Jacub's body from a distance. He waited a few minutes to make sure he did not move. Then, he called 911.

- 29 -

SCHNITZEL

Names
Tuesday, May 25, 2032, 8:30 p.m.

Schnitzel, the old man, and the woman walked down the small path in the Redwood forest. It was completely dark now, and the path was only lit sparingly by the blue light chains along the way.

Schnitzel noticed six glowing red eyes coming closer behind the dense shrubs that covered the forest floor. They smelled of coyote again. He growled, and the smell became less intense as the prairie wolves retreated, as they'd better. Next time, he would get one of them.

He heard some crushing twigs. It smelled of deer. One of the coyotes howled. More crushing twigs. The smell of deer and coyotes disappeared and was replaced with the stinking smell of a skunk. Schnitzel sneezed. This was awful.

The old man patted his head. "Come this way," he said.

They had reached the street again, and now headed to the left. The streetlamps were brighter here, and there were no wild animals around, as far as Schnitzel could tell.

"I wish I could just talk with her one last time," the woman said. "There are so many things I would like to tell her. Like how much I loved her."

"She knew that," the man said.

"Why do we send our children to these universities?" the woman said. "They end up millions of miles away. In the best-case scenario, they call you once in a while because they need something. In the worst-case scenario, they become busy and successful, and you hardly hear of them again, let alone see them in person. Or, as in our case, they end up dead."

"Usually, children outlive their parents. I just wanted her to be well-off when we weren't around anymore."

Tears glistened on the woman's face. "I was so proud of her."

The man took her hand. "Do you think we will see her again?"

"Do you mean in heaven?" the woman asked. "Of course, we will!"

They were interrupted by a sharp cry and a dull sound. Schnitzel's head and ears went up, and he noticed a suffocating smell of human blood coming down the street towards him. This was a village of death!

The couple looked down the street. "What was that?" the man said.

"I'm not sure," the woman responded. "I think it came from the building over there." She pointed at the SUEC research building.

The man stepped forward, his hand flat above his eyebrows. "I can't see anything," he said.

"Perhaps it was another coyote. There are so many wild animals around here. It's a miracle that our Nia was never attacked."

Schnitzel looked at them with pity. These humans were completely clueless. It was a miracle how they survived a single day—probably only due to the excellent protection by their canine friends. He growled and ran towards the source of the blood to find out what this was about.

"Hey, stay here," the old man shouted. He ran after the dog, but Schnitzel was faster, and he could see better at night than the old man.

There was a human body on the ground in front of the research building. Schnitzel stopped at the fence that separated the research building from the street. How could he get through? There was an entrance a few meters down the road, but he felt a jerk at his neck. The old man had grabbed his collar and was holding him back.

The man looked at the body and then up to the roof of the building. Something was moving there. Schnitzel could see that there was a human on the roof. He barked.

"Shush," the man mumbled. The full moon and lamps around the building provided enough light for him to see the man on the roof as well. He turned around quickly, pulling Schnitzel with him. "Let's go," he said. "We don't want to get in trouble—or worse."

He produced another cookie from his pocket, and Schnitzel decided to comply. He was really hungry, and nobody was threatening them.

They walked back to the woman. "What was that?" she asked.

"I believe a man fell from the building. He's dead."

"What?"

"There was another man on the roof."

"Oh, my god! Do you think he pushed him?"

"Perhaps it was an accident. Or not. I don't know."

"Did the man on the roof see you?"

"He seemed to be busy getting down. I don't believe he saw me. But I'm not sure. The dog barked."

"Are we in danger?"

"Don't worry. I have my gun here." He pointed at his jacket. "I will defend us if need be. And if this was Nia's murderer, then I will bring him down."

"Don't do anything stupid!" The woman waved her index finger at the man. "I cannot lose you too! Hopefully, Nia's body will be released tomorrow, and then we will leave this godforsaken place!"

They turned around and continued their walk down the street, albeit more quickly than before. The man did not let go of Schnitzel's collar. After a few more minutes, they reached a tall building with large glass double doors and an armada of bicycles in the front. The man opened the door. A warm breeze and an avalanche of different smells came at Schnitzel. Probably hundreds of humans lived here. And several other dogs. He liked it here.

The three stepped into the building and walked up the stairs and down a long hallway. The man opened a door at the end. It led into a small apartment. They entered a small foyer that led into a living room with a large couch and a fluffy carpet. It felt very soft under Schnitzel's paws. The woman turned the lights on, and the man led go of Schnitzel's collar.

Schnitzel put his muzzle into the air. No other dogs were here, but Nia's smell was everywhere. This was her cave.

Schnitzel walked around. No food in the living room. To the left was a small bedroom with an adjacent bathroom. The door was closed. Good. He had no interest in seeing another bathroom any time soon. To their right was a small kitchen that emitted a delicious smell. Schnitzel entered. Fresh bread was on the counter. Schnitzel sat down on the kitchen floor, nose up to the table, flaunting his most appealing posture. The women laughed. "You are hungry, aren't you?"

Schnitzel licked his lips. The man chuckled. "Don't spoil him." He reached for Schnitzel's collar again, but Schnitzel jumped to the side. The man was too slow to follow. He would not get him if Schnitzel did not want him to.

The woman opened a drawer, produced a knife, got the bread, and cut off a big slice. To Schnitzel's delight, she then opened the refrigerator and produced a terrific-smelling meaty spread. She added some to the bread, bent down, and offered it to Schnitzel. Schnitzel sniffed it carefully, considering his previous experience with the sandwich. But both this woman and her bread smelled good. Schnitzel took it and chewed it with delight.

The man had approached him from behind. He suddenly grabbed his collar and pulled the memory stick off. Schnitzel looked at him, chewing. *That was probably okay. The humans had paid their dues.*

The woman put water into a plastic bowl and placed it on the floor. Schnitzel drank carefully. The water reminded him of the bathtub. A shiver ran down his spine. He looked at the woman. She smiled. Was he safe now? She seemed trustworthy.

Schnitzel walked over to the fluffy carpet. He turned around himself four times to flatten it and then laid down. *What a day. Time for a nap.*

The man sat down on the couch beside him, fetched the laptop from the coffee table, and placed it on his thighs. He put the memory stick into the computer and typed something on the keyboard. The woman sat down beside him. Schnitzel observed them through half-open eyes, his erect ears adjusting to the typing noise like triangular satellite dishes.

"Look at this," the man said. Schnitzel looked up. More bread? But the man was looking at the woman. "There is a file with the name *fambly*. That is patois!"

"How peculiar," the woman said. "Most of the people here are either white or Asian. Who would speak a Caribbean dialect here?"

"Nia?" the man said.

"Do you really think we've met a random dog here on campus who is carrying a message from Nia to us? That would be too much of a coincidence."

"Perhaps not. If the dog knew Nia, he might have somehow recognized that we belong to her."

The woman patted Schnitzel's head. He looked up at her with his soft and kind eyes. "Perhaps," she said. Then she looked at the man. "What is on the *fambly* file, anyways?"

The man opened the file and scrolled through it. "It is a list of patients who had an infection and were successfully treated. I assume it is some research project from SUEC. Perhaps the researcher tested a new drug that treats infections."

The woman looked at the list over his shoulder.

Patient Number	IVF	Infection	Therapy response
1	+	Coccidiomycosis	resolved
2	+	Pneumococcus pneumonia	resolved
3	+	Tuberculosis	resolved
4	+	Pneumococcus pneumonia	resolved
5	+	COVID-19	resolved
6	+	COVID-19	resolved
7	+	COVID-19	resolved
8	+	COVID-19	resolved
9	+	Tuberculosis	resolved
10	+	Tuberculosis	resolved
11	+	Tuberculosis	resolved
12	+	Mucormycosis	resolved
13	+	Mucormycosis	resolved
14	+	Staphylococcus	resolved
15	+	*Pneumocystis jiroveci pneumonia*	resolved
16	+	Aspergillus	resolved
17	+	E. coli - pyelonephritis	resolved
18	+	E. coli - pyelonephritis	resolved
19	+	E. coli - hemolytic uremic syndrome	resolved
20	+	E. coli - enteritis	resolved
21	+	Salmonella pancreatitis	resolved
22	+	Helicobacter pylori gastritis	resolved

"And all patients had IVF?" she asked.

"What does that mean?

"In vitro fertilization."

"Do you mean they had assistance to conceive a child?

"Maybe. Or the patients themselves were conceived by IVF."

"Like Nia?"

"Yes, like Nia. And perhaps Nia was one of these patients. Do you remember she had that nasty pneumonia last year? But she recovered completely."

"Well, most patients recover from their pneumonia."

"Not all of them. Remember, many patients with COVID developed infections over and over again. And your sister had tuberculosis and has had problems exercising since then."

"Nia worked in the lab of an infectious-disease researcher. Perhaps they were testing a new drug that treats infections."

"She never mentioned anything like that."

"Perhaps it was a secret."

They both looked at the list of patients.

"So, all of these patients had an infection," the woman said. "The types of infection varied. For example, some had COVID, and others has tuberculosis. It seems that all of them were successfully treated, though. If SUEC researchers were testing a new drug, could it treat any infection? I'm not sure if that is possible."

"Perhaps that's what was so unique about it. And Nia collected all the data."

"But then why would anybody shoot her? If she was part of the research team, they would need her to analyze the results."

The man shook his head. "I don't know how that could make sense. I think we're still missing something. Today, I recorded a conversation with Nia's research supervisor and the FBI agent. The researcher confessed that she was guilty, but then she only said that she'd cursed Nia."

"Nia was a rebel. If she died every time someone cursed her, she would have been long-dead already."

The man chuckled. "Do you remember when she got that watercolor tattoo on her shoulder?"

The woman sighed. "I was so mad! Why would she disfigure her spotless skin like that?"

"It was a Chinese character. And she told you that it translated to *I love you, mom*."

"Of course, it didn't. It was the sign for *courage*." Tears welled up in the woman's eyes and rolled down her face, trickling down her chin and landing on Schnitzel's right ear. He looked up, rose on his paws, and put his big head on her lap.

"You are one of a kind," she said with a broken voice, patting his head.

The man clicked on the trackpad of the computer. "There is another file," he said.

- 30 -

TERREL

The Interview
Wednesday, May 25, 2033, 8:30 p.m.

Terrel Wright's eVTOL aircraft landed on the helipad of SUEC hospital. In the distance, the sun had plunged into the evening fog, leaving a tapestry of hazy pink behind the modern limestone building.

Terrel walked swiftly to the entrance of the ER. The sliding glass doors opened promptly and shut behind him. An elderly lady at the reception desk looked him up and down through gold wire-framed glasses. He showed her his FBI ID and asked for Ingrid.

She walked him down a sterile white hallway that smelled of disinfectant. A mechanical voice called out medical codes through speakers at the ceiling. A nurse with an elderly man in a squeaking wheelchair passed by. They stopped at a door flanked by an SUEC security guard. Terrel showed his ID again, and the guard opened the door for him.

Terrel stepped into a small patient room. He saw Ingrid lying in the bed in front of him with a big bandage around her left hand and an infusion connected to her right arm. Heinz was sitting beside her, holding her hand. He jumped up when he saw Terrel. "Agent Wright, it's good to see you! Did you find my dog?" he asked.

"My colleague found a German Shepherd in an apartment on the SUEC campus. We have reason to believe that this is your dog, but I'm afraid on my way here, I got a text message that he ran away."

"Oh, my god! Do you know where he went?"

"He must be somewhere on the SUEC campus."

Heinz turned to Ingrid. "Ingrid, I have to go to the campus right away. I need to find Schnitzel. You're in good hands now."

She smiled at him. "Of course! Go get your dog, Heinzi!"

He leaned over to her and squeezed her hand. "I will be back as soon as possible."

Terrel interrupted. "I actually came here to see Mrs. Maulvi."

Heinz looked at Terrel. "Ingrid was kidnapped. Fortunately, she managed to escape. She suffered severe injuries, and just got an MRI scan. We don't know the result yet."

"Aren't you in medical care here as well, Mr. Tremblay?"

"I was discharged an hour ago. When I wanted to leave, Ingrid was brought in. I was terrified when I heard that she had been kidnapped. I wanted to make sure she was okay."

Ingrid cleared her throat. "Don't worry about me, Heinz. I'm in the best hospital in the world here. And Agent Wright will make sure that I'm safe, right?" She raised her gaze to Terrel with a look of wide-eyed innocence.

Terrel pointed at the door. "There is an SUEC security guard at your door, Mrs. Maulvi. He will make sure that nobody enters or leaves this room without permission. I'm here because I investigate threats to the national security of the United States. I have a few questions for you about the recent incidents."

Ingrid nodded. "Of course. I'm at your service, Agent Wright. Thank you for placing a security guard at my door."

Terrel sighed. The security guard was there to make sure Ingrid could not run away, but there was no need to clarify that now. He looked at Heinz. "Mr. Tremblay, if you feel well enough, please go to the SUEC campus and look for your dog. I would like to talk with Mrs. Maulvi in private."

"Of course," Heinz said. "If Schnitzel is there, I will find him!"

"The SUEC security team is also looking for him. He was last seen close to the SUEC research building, but then he disappeared."

Heinz leaned towards Ingrid and kissed her forehead. "Stay safe." Then, he turned around and left the room.

Terrel waited until Heinz had closed the door behind him. Then, he turned back to Ingrid. "Ingrid, it has come to our attention that you hired an exotic dancer a couple of weeks ago."

Ingrid raised her eyebrows. "Is that a crime of national interest?"

"Well, this person is linked to a federal felony."

She shrugged. "I have nothing to do with that. I hired him for a bachelor party; you can check that."

"The pay was much higher than for a standard gig."

"Well, what can I say? We paid extra for discretion."

"The delicate part here is that this person was found dead last night."

"Oh, that is horrible." Ingrid looked at him with blank expression. "Was he killed as well?

"We don't know that yet. He fell from his balcony."

"I am so sorry. Accidents happen."

They stared at each other. She was clearly lying.

And there was nothing he could do about it.

Someone knocked at the door, and a nurse came in—the same nurse whom Terrell had met earlier in Heinz's room. She looked at him in surprise. "Hello, Mr. Wright. Are you interviewing all of our patients today?"

"No, only the ones who can provide information about criminal activities."

"Well, this is a hospital, not a train station. Our patients here need rest." She walked to Ingrid and checked the infusion pump with the antibiotics, then reached for Ingrid's wrist and palpated her pulse. She looked up at Terrel. "Well, Mrs. Maulvi's heart rate is far too high. Is this because of your discussions of criminal activities?"

So, Ingrid was anxious after all. She had just played unconcerned. Terrel shrugged. "I don't know. Perhaps Mrs. Maulvi can enlighten us?"

Ingrid evaded his gaze and looked at the nurse. "Agent Wright just told me that another man might have been murdered. Of course, I am disturbed by that."

The nurse looked at Terrel with a disapproving gaze. "Mr. Wright, I would appreciate it if you could avoid upsetting my patient."

"No worries," he responded. "I only have a few more questions, and then I will be gone."

"Please try to be time-efficient. I will check back on my patient in a few minutes." The nurse turned around and left the room.

There was silence for a moment.

Ingrid straightened her bedlinen with her uninjured hand. "I was just kidnapped," she said. "Are you not concerned about me?"

"Of course, I'm concerned about your safety, Ingrid. That's why I'm here." Terrel knew that she was lying about the exotic dancer. She knew about his death.

But he would play along. Persistence would get some information out of her eventually. "Perhaps you can tell me what happened to *you* this morning?" he asked.

Ingrid sighed. "Well, I don't remember that much. I lost consciousness, like Heinz. I woke up in an apartment with my arms and feet tied. I managed to free myself and ran for the door. There was an angry dog in the room, and it bit me." Ingrid held up her hand and lifted a bandaged foot. "I made it through the door and closed it. Then I ran to the street, and a police officer picked me up."

This was the most fantastic story Terrel had heard in a long time. "Why would anybody kidnap you?" he asked.

"I have no idea," Ingrid said with an upturned gaze.

"Do you think that this incident had any connection to Nia Johnes's death?"

"I don't know. You tell me."

"We found out that Nia, you, and Heinz are related."

"Yes, we are half-siblings."

"You didn't mention this when we talked earlier today."

"Well, it's private information. I didn't think that anybody would shoot me because I am Nia's sister."

"And Oliver Stuart Robinson is your father?"

"Yes, he is!" she said with a proud voice.

"He was a sperm donor? How did you get that information? It is usually kept confidential," Terrel asked.

"My mother told me the donor number. I looked it up in the California donor registry and found that my father was a professor. I had just finished my PhD and was having difficulties finding a postdoctoral fellowship position. No connections, you know. I took all my savings and hired a private investigator. He found out that it was Oliver. I could not believe it at first. It was an amazing revelation."

"Amazing?"

"Yeah. My other father—the man who raised me—had Huntington's disease, a serious inherited disease that leads to involuntary jerking movements and personality changes. He died during the COVID pandemic. For all my life, I was terrified that I had inherited his illness. Then, I found out that my actual father was a world-famous professor. Not only did I not inherit the Huntington's gene, I had been given genes from one of the smartest men on the planet. I was so relieved and excited! I love science!"

"And you revealed your discovery to Dr. Robinson?"

"Yes, I met with Oliver and told him that I knew that I was his daughter. He was as delighted as I was. He has other children, but none of them were interested in his research, and I had trained in exactly his field. He offered me a position in his lab."

"Did other lab members know that you're his daughter?"

"No, we kept it private. Oliver wants me to take over the lab one day. That would be more difficult if it were known that we're related."

"Heinz is Dr. Robinson's son as well?"

"Yes, he is, but Oliver asked me to keep this private as well. He could sue me if I revealed it without his permission. So, I kept my mouth shut. Heinz only knows that the three of us are diblings."

"Nia, you, and Heinz got to know each other?"

"We got to know each other at a dibling party."

"And then you all started working at SUEC?"

"After meeting Oliver, I started working there first. Heinz had only recently moved to San Francisco. I forwarded him a job ad from SUEC, and he got the job. Oliver forwarded Nia's CV to Cristina. Nia's skills were a great fit for Cristina's lab, and she hired her."

"And Nia knew that Dr. Robinson was her father?"

"She did not know that when Cristina hired her, but she found it out recently. Unlike me, she was not happy about it. She wanted to report Oliver to the University for playing with her genes. But it was not playing—he had just donated genes that would make his offspring stronger. I am very grateful for that."

"Jacub saw you arguing with Nia the night before she died. Was that what you argued about?"

"Yes. Nia threatened us, saying that she wanted to report Oliver. I told her to drop it. This could jeopardize our entire lab—and my future career. But she wouldn't listen!"

"And then you killed her?"

"I told you my whole life, and you are accusing me again?" Ingrid exclaimed with a high-pitched voice. "I did not do anything. I am the victim here! I was kidnapped!"

Terrel remained unimpressed. This woman was a serial liar—the pretended gun shot, the kidnapping story, the way she evaded his gaze. Perhaps some parts of her story were true, but it was hard to tell which ones. "So, Dr. Robinson killed Nia?" he asked.

Ingrid raised her hands. "Oliver is the sweetest man on the planet. He would never hurt anyone!"

"So, who did it?"

"Am I the FBI?"

Terrel was starting to lose his patience. "Ingrid, your story does not make sense. You said that you were kidnapped in broad daylight. But there are no witnesses who can confirm your story."

"Well, the kidnapper obviously got away. If someone had seen them, they would not have been able to bring me to that apartment."

"You said that your hands and feet were tied, but there are no marks on your wrists or ankles." Terrel pointed at her hands.

"It was a shawl or something. It didn't leave any marks. That dog bit me. That you can see, right?" She held up her bandaged hand.

"Yes, a dog bit you, but we do not know the circumstances. How can you explain that that same dog was stuffed into a suitcase and nearly drowned?"

"I have no idea. That sounds horrible." She clutched her free hand to her chest. "I think my heart might start racing again."

"Ingrid, did you know that not cooperating with the FBI is a felony?"

"I'm telling you nothing but the truth!" Ingrid raised her voice. "Why would you not believe me? You're making me really uncomfortable here. Do you have a problem with women? I will make a complaint that you treated me disrespectfully."

They stared at each other in mutual frustration.

Terrel's cell phone rang. "We will talk again, Ingrid," he said calmly. Then, he turned around and walked out of the room.

Outside, he answered the phone. "FBI special Agent Terrel Wright here."

"Hello, Terrel, this is Lamong. We were just informed that Jacub Bezdomny fell from the roof of the SUEC research building. He's dead."

"I'm on my way. Did the microphone on his lapel button record anything unusual?"

"Well, we recorded a conversation where an SUEC security guard informed Dr. Stuart Robinson that Ingrid Maulvi spiked someone's drink some time ago. That person ended up in the ER and was diagnosed with an infection."

All discoveries in this case seemed to be linked to Ingrid Maulvi.

"Interesting," Terrel said. "Anything else?"

"Dr. Stuart Robinson asked Jacub to check the antenna on the roof. So, he sent him there. But he was also the one who called 911."

"Okay. I'll talk with him first."

Lamong cleared his throat. "Well, there's something else. Agent Angus Weber just arrived, and he would like to talk with you as well."

Terrel heard some rustling noises. Then, he heard his boss's voice. "Hello, Terrel."

"Hello, Angus. What's the matter? Why are you on campus?"

"Well, earlier today, Dr. Stuart Robinson made a complaint that the FBI is not doing a good enough job on this case."

"Did he complain about me specifically?"

"Sort of. Yes. Listen, I have every confidence in you, Terrel. But I don't want your career to get hurt by complaints from SUEC. I will join you in the investigation. Then, Dr. Robinson can complain about both of us if he's not happy."

Terrel sighed. Of course, if he was successful, the success would be attributed to his boss as well. It wouldn't be the first time. The black man did the work, but the white man received the accolades.

Angus was a great mentor. It was not his fault. It was the system. And it wasn't as if he had a choice here.

"Okay. Should we meet at the eVTOL landing pad at SUEC?"

"Yes, that's a good idea. See you there."

- 31 -

LILI

Osteomyelitis
Wednesday, May 25, 2033, 8:30 p.m.

Lili had reviewed the abstract of her student Ying, sent the edited version back to him, and was just getting ready to leave her office when her cell phone rang. It was the radiology resident. "Hello, Lili. I'm sorry to bother you again. I know you were up last night, but you're on call this whole week, right?"

"Yes, I am."

"Are you still on campus?"

"I'm at the SUEC research center. I was just getting ready to drive home. What's the matter?"

"Well, one of the patients in the ER just got an MRI of the hand and foot after a dog bite. There are two police officers here, and they want an overread by an attending."

"No problem. I have a PACS workstation here. Give me just a minute." Lili sat down at the desk and turned on her computer. "What is the medical record number of the patient?"

The resident dictated the patient number.

"Ingrid Maulvi?" Lili exclaimed. "What happened to her?"

"You know her? She's an SUEC employee, right?"

"Yes, I know her. In fact, I talked with her this morning. She'd encountered an injury to her arm then." She did not want to mention that Ingrid had been shot at. "What happened to her now?"

"I'm afraid I didn't talk with her, and there isn't much information in her file," the resident responded. "The only thing I know is that she was bitten by a dog, and two police officers here want to know the degree of the injury for the incident report."

"Did Ingrid agree to release that information?"

"Yes, she signed a release form."

"Okay, let me have a look." Lili opened the images in the picture archiving computer system. She looked at the images of the hand first and explained the findings to the resident. "The MRI scan shows a deep soft tissue laceration of the index finger and a large effusion of the distal interphalangeal joint. The joint surfaces are very irregular. There is abnormal contrast-enhancement of the affected joint and adjacent bone marrow of the mid and end phalanx. This is severe septic arthritis with associated osteomyelitis, an infection of the joint and adjacent bones."

"The patient was bitten by a dog."

"Yes, you can see the bite marks in the skin. The finger is quite swollen. This is a serious infection and needs urgent intravenous antibiotic treatment. It can deteriorate very fast."

"Thank you. I'm really glad that you looked at the images right away. Can you please also have a look at the images of the foot as well?"

"Of course!" Lili brought up the images of the foot. "These look very similar to the images of the hand," she said. "You now know what to look for. Tell me what you see."

The resident cleared her throat. "Well, the MRI scan demonstrates an effusion in the distal interphalangeal joint of the fourth toe with surrounding soft tissue swelling. There is marked contrast enhancement of the joint and adjacent bone marrow. This is septic arthritis with associated osteomyelitis."

"Exactly. The most common germ that leads to an infection after a dog bite is *Pasteurella canis*. Again, this patient needs immediate antibiotic treatment."

"Thanks! I feel confident to make this diagnosis next time."

"Great. The imaging findings may be more subtle in other cases, but now you know what to look for."

"Yes! I will inform the police officers and call the clinical team right away so that they can start the appropriate treatment."

"Okay. Have a good evening."

"You too! I hope I don't have to call you again today."

"No worries. You can call me anytime."

Lili sighed. She felt exhausted. The work never stopped. Hopefully, she could enjoy an uninterrupted late dinner with her husband Mark tonight.

She turned her computer off, grabbed her laptop bag, and left the building. The sun had set, and the patio in front of the research building was illuminated by flickering solar torches. The rose bushes in front of the building emanated a sweet fragrance, and the tall eucalyptus trees to her right were rustling in the evening breeze.

As Lili walked down the path to the street, she saw a large crowd in front of the research building to her left. A police officer was blocking the gate to the street. *I've had enough for today*, Lili thought as she walked briskly towards him. *Whatever this is, I'm not interested.* She did not look to the crowd. She wanted to get out of here.

She tried to pass the police officer, but he stepped in front of her, extending both arms. "Hello, miss. Did you just come out of this building?"

Lili pointed back at the research building. "Do you mean the SUEC research building? Yes, I work here."

"Can you please step aside? We have to interrogate everyone on the property."

Oh, no. What is this? "Why? What happened?"

Lili looked around. There were several police officers and SUEC security guards to her left. She heard the siren of an arriving ambulance. It stopped with squeaking wheels. Two paramedics jumped out and ran to the group in front of the building. The guards stepped aside to make space for the arriving medical team, and Lili could see a body on the floor—a man in a silver suit in a lake of dark-red blood. "Is that Jacub?" she cried. She wanted to run towards the body.

"Please step back, ma'am." The police officer held his arm in front of her.

One of the paramedics knelt down, palpated the man's pulse, inspected his head, and then stepped back. "He's dead," he said loud and clear.

Lili felt dizzy. She sat down on the lawn beside the path. Her chest felt tight. It was hard to breathe. She pulled out her cell phone. The police officer looked wary. "Can I call my husband?" she asked.

"Of course," he responded.

A man separated from the group around the dead man and came towards them. Lili looked up. It was Dr. Robinson. *That man again.* She put down the phone.

"Lili, what are you doing here at this late hour?" he asked.

"I had to finish some work," she said coldly.

"You were in the building?" he asked with raised eyebrows.

The policeman looked alerted.

"Yes. Remember, we met here this afternoon?" Lili raised her voice. *What sick game is he playing this time?*

"I saw you this afternoon. But that was more than two hours ago. Were you here since then?"

"As I said, I had to finish some work. Why do you care?"

"Well, our building manager just fell of the roof. We don't know if he fell or if he was pushed, so everyone who was in the building at the time of the incident is a suspect."

"You mean to imply that *I* could be a suspect for a murder?"

The police officer looked at Lili and made a note in his notebook.

This is too much. She clenched her fists. "Well, I was on the phone with the radiology resident to review a case."

"For two hours?" Dr. Robinson said calmly.

Lili clenched her fists. "Before that, I reviewed an urgent abstract that's due tonight of one of my students."

"You reviewed abstracts just a few hours before the deadline? Do you have a witness for that?"

Lili blushed. "What were *you* doing during the last two hours, Dr. Robinson?"

The police officer raised his hands. "Please calm down, folks. Here comes the cavalry." He pointed to the street, where a self-driving SUEC electric vehicle had just stopped.

Agent Terrel Wright and Angus Weber stepped out and walked towards the man on the ground.

- 32 -

ANNYA

The Revelation
Wednesday, May 25, 2033, 8:30 p.m.

Annya had brought the semen samples to the genetics lab at SUEC hospital. Fortunately, Charles, the chief technician, was on service. He agreed to analyze the samples right away, no questions asked. It would take about two hours.

Hopefully, she had done the right thing here. If she could shine light on the Nia case, everyone would be grateful. But if this was a red herring, then she and Cristina would get in trouble. Dr. Robinson would probably file a complaint either way. And retaliate.

But she was too old to be intimidated by bullies. *If he wants to fire me, I will happily hand over my shifts,* she thought. But he probably couldn't. The hospital would brush it over. She was too valuable, too experienced, and she didn't mind working around the clock. The younger generation had different expectations about work–life balance. The hospital would have to hire two, perhaps three physicians to replace her when she retired one day.

Annya walked over to the ER to see if she could help out there while waiting for the results from the genetics lab. It was not her shift, but she was the division chief here, so she felt responsible.

She walked down the long, narrow, neon-lit hallway, which was less busy than earlier today, and stepped aside to make room for a beeping robot that was cleaning the linoleum floor. It smelled of chlorine. The surgery resident rushed by, adjusting his face mask, not taking notice of her. He was possibly on his way to the OR. She passed a man who leaned down to console a crying girl with a splint on her right arm.

How many times had she seen the cycle of pain, suffering, and consolation? She did not remember.

As she approached the main ER hub, Annya was surprised to see a SUEC guard at the entrance of one of the exam rooms. What was he guarding in her ER?

She showed him her physician ID and went in. In the bed in front of her was Ingrid. Her face was pale, her eyes were closed, her long dark hair was scattered around her head, and her chest was gently moving up and down. She was sleeping. Her left arm was wrapped in a bandage, and her right arm was connected to an infusion pump. Annya stepped closer. Antibiotics.

She watched Ingrid for a while. She looked so innocent and peaceful, but this young woman had fabricated an assault and framed Cristina. Who knew what else she was capable of?

Ingrid opened her eyes and looked at Annya. Was there a hint of surprise in her gaze? It was hard to tell. Her eyebrows and forehead were frozen, as usual. "Hello, Dr. Segond," she said. "What brings you here?"

"I work here, Ingrid. I could ask you the same question."

"I was kidnapped and bitten by a dog." She held up her arm, which ended in a big bandage ball.

"Kidnapped by Cristina Walker-Díaz?"

"I suppose. I was drugged and woke up in her apartment. I escaped."

Who would believe this fantastic story? Ingrid was lying in the hospital bed like a dying princess. Annya quickly got annoyed with this theater.

"Cut the crap, Ingrid. Cristina has multiple witnesses who can confirm that she was in the SUEC research building all day long. Your story does not hold up."

"Perhaps she hired someone to do the job."

"And she did that because?"

"I don't know. You tell me."

Annya inhaled deeply. "Sure, I'll tell you what I think, Ingrid. I received a notification about a new patent that Dr. Stuart Robinson filed—a new approach to map multiple genes of sperms, oocytes, and embryos. I have to admit, it is quite genius. Active manipulation of the genome is prohibited, but he just provides genetic profiling with unprecedented detail. It does not say so in the patent, but it is obvious that he could create designer babies. He is already screening embryos for genetic diseases before their implantation. Why not check a few other genes while he's at it? Gender, eye color, hair color, complexion, athletic ability, intelligence, and the ability to fight off infections. He can provide a gene map of multiple embryos, and the customer can choose their favorite."

Ingrid smiled. "Oliver and I are geniuses indeed."

"You helped him with this work?

"I am his right hand. One day, I will take over the lab."

"Is that what he promised you? Do you know what else that genius did?"

"Ignored your negative aura?"

"He did not include you on the patent, Ingrid."

Ingrid stared at Annya. *That* had been news to her. Her eyebrows slowly moved together. Annya looked at her with fascination. She had thought that Ingrid's entire forehead was paralyzed. It was not. Her eyebrows could move a little. "You are lying!" Ingrid screamed.

Annya pulled her smart phone out of her pocket, opened the patent file, and handed it to Ingrid. "See for yourself. The patent was published today."

Ingrid snatched the phone from her and flipped through the patent document with her big bandaged hand, staring at the screen.

"This must be a mistake," she said with a creaking voice.

"He is using you, Ingrid," Annya said calmly.

Ingrid looked up at her, tears welling up in her eyes. "I'm sure he can explain. Oliver is my father, and he is looking out for me!"

Annya looked at her with pity. Ingrid reminded her of her younger self. She, too, had fallen in love with a psychopath as a young woman. And she, too, had been hurt. "I'm sorry that you were used, Ingrid," she repeated.

She had to let the information sink in. Acceptance would come eventually, and then Ingrid would cooperate. Hopefully.

"I was *not* used!" Ingrid responded, curling her lips. "And this is not your business, anyways. You are a physician, not a preacher. And you are doing a shitty job here. You did not bother to check my hand."

"I did check it when I came in, Ingrid. You were bitten by a dog. You got antibiotics, and the chart above your bed shows that you got a tetanus vaccine. Your injury is taken care of."

"So, why are you talking smack about Oliver? Are you jealous? Go away!" Ingrid threw the cell phone at Annya.

With a quick leap, Annya caught it with her right hand. The two women locked eyes. Then, Annya turned around and left the room.

Oliver was likely the mastermind behind Nia's death. And it was devastating that he had used this young woman to do the dirty work.

Annya walked back down the hallway to the ER hub. She had to wait for the results of the PCR analyses. Why not be useful in the meantime? Attending to patients' injuries and physical pain helped her to calm her own mind, to feel like she was making a difference. The smile of an elderly man whose chest pain had been treated, the hug of a mother whose son was resuscitated after a car crash. Helping the injured and forgotten to get back on their feet was intensely gratifying to her.

Annya's cell phone rang. "Hello?"

"Hi, Annya. This is Lamong from the FBI headquarters in San Francisco. Do you have a minute?"

"Sure. What's up?"

"We got intel that Ingrid Maulvi spiked the drinks of several young adults at dibling parties."

"What did she spike the drinks with?"

"Well, that's the interesting part—it seems that some of the victims got sick a few days later. We're wondering if she spiked the drinks with bacteria or other infectious agents."

"'Spiked the drinks with bacteria?' Why would she do that?"

"We have to find that out, but first, we would like to confirm that all victims did indeed develop an infection."

"And that's why you need my help?"

"Exactly. Could you please look up two patients for me? They were both patients at SUEC hospital."

"I assume you have a warrant?"

"Yes, I do. I forwarded it to your email address."

"Okay." Annya checked her phone and confirmed it. "Who are the patients?"

Lamong provided the medical record number of the first patient. Annya reviewed their medical file and imaging scans. "This is a thirty-year-old patient with severe pancreatitis. There is a CT scan that shows a swollen pancreas with diminished enhancement after contrast media injection. In addition, there is extensive ascites throughout the abdomen. A bacterial analysis demonstrated salmonella in the stool.

That is unusual. Most cases of pancreatitis occur due to an obstructing stone in the common bile duct."

"This patient's drink was spiked on January 12. When was the CT scan done?"

"January 16. So, the patient got sick a few days after the drink was spiked."

"I guess that confirms our theory."

Annya looked through the file. "It's also remarkable that this infection resolved completely within three weeks. That is unusual."

"Thanks, I will make a note of that. Can you have a look at the second patient as well?"

"Sure."

Lamong dictated the medical record number of the second patient. "This is a fifteen-year-old male."

"A minor? Ingrid spiked his drink as well?

"Yes, on March 1."

"Does she have no scruples?"

"Apparently not."

Annya shook her head as she flipped through the patient's file. "Unbelievable. There is a CT scan from March 3, two days later."

"What does it show?"

"There is marked swelling and edema of the gastric wall of the antrum, the lowermost part of the stomach. This is most likely gastritis. The note states that an endoscopy demonstrated helicobacter pylori as the underlying germ."

"Did the infection resolve as well?"

"Yes, it completely resolved within ten days."

"Remarkable! Thank you. This was very helpful."

"Do you know that Ingrid Maulvi is currently here in the hospital?"

"Yes, of course we know that. She's a person of interest, and we've placed her under observation. We have to collect more evidence before we can convict her."

"Do you think there's a mastermind behind these actions?"

"Possibly. We're looking into that as well."

"Okay. Let me know if you need any help."

"You've already helped us immensely, Annya. Thank you for your service."

Annya hung up and processed the information for a while. Then, she called Charles in the genetics lab. "Hi, Charles. Can you do me a favor?"

"Another one?"

"Yes and no—a related one. Can you please specifically look for infection-associated genes in the samples that I brought to you about an hour ago?"

"Do you have anything specific in mind?"

"One that I read about a few years ago was the *CCR5*-delta32 mutation. Perhaps start with that? But if you know any other infection-related genes, can you please check those as well?"

"Annya, looking at *CCR5*- delta32 will be at least an extra two hours."

"Please. It is really important."

He sighed. "If you hadn't saved me when I came to the ER with a fractured shoulder, I would say no. I'll get it for you, professor, but then, we are even."

"Of course, Charles. Thank you!"

- 33 -

SCHNITZEL

The Files
Wednesday, May 25, 2033, 8:30 p.m.

Mrs. Johnes patted Schnitzel's head. He looked up at her with his big eyes, snuffling at her hand with his wet nose, his tail wagging. Perhaps there was an opportunity here to get a treat.

On the couch beside her, her husband did not react at all. He continued to stare at the laptop computer on his lap. Neither of them offered him food. That was disappointing. That bread had been an appetizer at most. Did they not know that a German Shepherd needed more food? Where was the main course?

The woman scratched him behind his right ear. Schnitzel liked that. He tried to be patient. They had to eat eventually.

"Look at this," the man said.

"What is it?" the woman asked.

"This is Nia's birth certificate!"

The woman leaned over and stared at the screen. "My goodness!"

"And there is a letter from the donor sibling registry addressed to Nia Johnes!"

"It is her memory stick indeed!" The woman grabbed Schnitzel's head with both hands and kissed his forehead. He grunted with approval. *More, please.*

But the woman had already turned her attention back to the screen. "What does it say?" she asked.

"It informs her that she has two half-siblings: Dr. Ingrid Maulvi and Mr. Heinz Tremblay."

"Oh! Nia always wanted to have a sister or a brother. Why did she not tell us about it?"

The man shrugged.

The woman looked over his shoulder. "There is another note here that they all work at SUEC. What a weird coincidence."

"I assume they got to know each other first and then looked for a job at the same institution," the man said. "There is another file here with medical images and a list of patients. Looks like they all had an infection of some type, and they all recovered."

"Perhaps they were testing a new drug. What is that?" The woman pointed at a small icon under the patient list.

"It's a voice memo," the man explained. I recorded some on my new iPhone today. It's really easy. You just turn it on and place it close to the people you want to listen in on."

"Can you turn it on?"

The man double-clicked it. They heard distant footsteps. Then, two women greeted each other.

"That is Nia's voice!" the woman exclaimed. "I can't believe it!" Tears streamed down her cheeks, seemingly unstoppable.

Schnitzel got up and licked her hands. She did not react but stared at the computer.

The man turned up the sound. They heard Nia's voice. "Hey, Ingrid, I know what you're up to. You're selecting babies for IVF who have genes that make them resistant to infections. That is illegal."

Another woman answered. "You should be thankful, Nia! You're stronger than most people. I only got one of the mutations, but you got both. We are part of a new generation of humans!"

"You have no right to play with other people's genes, Ingrid. There can be unintended consequences. For example, there have been reports that people who have double mutations of the CCR5 gene live less long than other people."

"That is a solvable problem. We only need enough data to map the effects. Then, people in the future can choose which genes they want."

"Which genes they want for their *baby*. You are not curing a genetic disease. You're playing with perfectly healthy embryos."

"Well, look at me. I have suffered paralysis of my *face* due to COVID, despite my single CCR5 gene mutation. We are learning fast. You have two mutations and recovered completely from your pneumonia. Any side effects can be addressed. Or we can find even better genes."

"You will *not* do that. I'll report you and your shady business!"

"Go ahead. Inform Oliver. He'll crush you in a heartbeat!"

"I will go to the police!"

The tape ended. Mrs. Johnes looked at her husband. "This is evidence. We have to bring it to the police now, and they can arrest these people."

Mr. Johnes looked at her. "You heard the woman—this is big business. They probably bought off the police. And got Nia killed. If we go to the police, we might get killed as well."

"But they killed our daughter! You want to let them get away with that?"

"No. I will personally take care of this." The man jumped up from the couch. "She said Oliver would crush Nia in a heartbeat. Let's see what I can do about that."

"Don't do anything stupid," the woman pleaded. "Perhaps we can inform the FBI agent. He seemed trustworthy."

"What is he going to do in this swamp of corruption? If the others want to sweep Nia's death under the carpet, they will. But *I* will not accept that. I will seek justice!"

"We didn't look through all the files yet," the woman said. "Let's at least get all the information straight. We still don't know exactly what happened."

She patted the seat beside her. The man reluctantly sat down and looked back at the screen. "Here is another file from the California Cryobank. A table with donor numbers."

The woman looked over his shoulder. "These are sperm donors," she said.

"How do you know?" he asked.

"That's where we got our sperm donation from."

"There is a number circled—6548."

"I remember that number very well. It is from Nia's sperm donor."

The man stared at the table. It provided details about numbers of pregnancies derived from the donor, occupation, years of education, height, weight, hair color, hair texture, and race/ethnic origin.

"You chose a Caucasian sperm donor? An English man? Why would you do that? We are both Black Caribbeans."

"He was the only professor on the list. I wanted our child to be really smart. Intelligence and a good education are the best path out of poverty, you know that."

"We are not poor, and we are smart enough ourselves to raise a smart kid. Do you have prejudice against our own kind?"

"No, of course not. We *were* poor when we were thinking about having a child. You had just completed chemotherapy, and you wanted to go on with your life and have a family. But I was scared. I did not know how long you would survive and if I might be a single mother one day. I wanted the smartest donor on the list. He happened to be white. So what?"

"So, if you had the choice, you would choose a white husband?"

"Don't be silly. I love you with all of my heart." She hugged him tightly.

He leaned away from her. "What if our child would have been white? Did you want to embarrass me in front of everyone?" He looked at her with disgust.

Tears welled up in her eyes. "No, of course not, honey. The clinic offered pre-implantation diagnoses. They created several embryos, and I could choose one with the desired gender, hair color, and complexion."

"Unbelievable." The man gave her a cold look. "There is a donor number, name and address," he said. "The same number. 6548—Dr. Oliver Stuart Robinson. Who is that?"

"I think you already know," the woman said softly. "You could google him if you want to see what he looks like?"

The man copied the name and googled it. "I know him!" he exclaimed. "He works in the same building as Nia. He was interrogated by the FBI agent today. *That* is her biological father?"

"I guess so. I never met him," the woman said softly.

"Well, Nia knew. She worked in the same building! The only one who was in the dark was me!" he cried with an angry voice.

"I have no idea why Nia and this man worked in the same building," the women said. "I don't know how this came about."

"Well, I will find out!" the man shouted. "That is the building where we just saw a man falling from the roof. Or being pushed. There was another man on the roof. If Dr. Robinson is responsible for Nia's death, I swear I will kill him!" He smashed the laptop down on the coffee table and jumped up from the couch.

Schnitzel jumped up and growled. This was too much hostility. This man needed some discipline.

The man walked over to the entrance, threw on his jacket, reached into his pocket, produced a gun, and cocked it."

"Don't do anything stupid!" the woman cried. She jumped up from her seat as well.

"Don't try to stop me," he said with a grim tone. "You have insulted me enough today."

She froze, tears streaming down her face. Schnitzel felt the tension and started barking at the man.

He turned around and left, slamming the door behind him.

Schnitzel tried to follow the man, but the door smashed shut in front of his nuzzle. He scratched at the door and continued to bark uncontrollably.

"Stop!" The woman tried to pull him back by his collar—just like the woman who squeezed him into the suitcase. Schnitzel jumped around and snapped at her. The woman led go, stumbled backwards, and fell to the floor. She looked at him with wide-open eyes. *Fear.*

He felt remorse. He really did not want to scare her. But he had important business to do here.

Schnitzel jumped back at the door, trying to turn the doorknob with his paws. He could open Heinz's office door, but it had a longer door handle. This one was round. How did the humans open it? Schnitzel jumped up and tried to crack it open with his teeth. The door did not move.

The woman slowly got up and walked into the kitchen. After a minute, she re-emerged with a slice of bread. Schnitzel looked back at her, his head tilted. "Sit!" she said calmly.

Schnitzel complied, directing his nuzzle to the bread. There was something meaty on it. It smelled too good to ignore.

Schnitzel wagged his tail. The woman handed it to him. He gladly accepted and swallowed it in one gulp.

She reached for the door and opened it. "Find him," she said.

Schnitzel jumped up and raced down the hallway, following the scent of the angry man.

- 34 -

TERREL

The Corps
Wednesday, May 25, 2033, 9:00 p.m.

FBI Special Agents Terrel Wright and Angus Weber walked towards the corpse in front of the SUEC research building. There were about twenty SUEC security guards with flashlights swirling around the octagonal limestone structure and the adjacent park. Most of them were walking in, on, and around the building, collecting evidence. Two guards were securing the premises with tape while two others guarded the corpse, two more held spectators back, and one interviewed SUEC employees who were exiting the building.

Terrel looked over his shoulder to two women who were sitting on a bench on the porch, talking with the SUEC guard. One of them was Lili. He waved. She waved back. Lili was an excellent observer. Perhaps she had noticed something.

But he had to check on the dead man first.

Angus had reached the corpse first. He knelt beside him and inspected him carefully. The man was lying on his back in a lake of blood on the brick path that surrounded the building.

Terrel recognized the man immediately. His occiput was smashed to pieces, but his face was surprisingly well-preserved. It was pale, motionless, frozen in a scream. "This is Jacub Bezdomny, the building manager," he said.

Jacub's lifeless green eyes stared at them. Terrel closed them with a gloved hand. "Goodbye, my friend," he murmured.

"Did you know him?" Angus asked.

Terrel wiped away a tear from the corner of his eye. "We had arrested him earlier today as a possible suspect," he said. "I found a gun in his office. Our forensics team confirmed that it was the gun that killed Nia, and his fingerprints were on it. But they also found out that these were old fingerprints—he had cut his finger shortly before Nia's death, and the new fingerprint with the cut was not on the gun. Someone had tried to frame him."

Angus looked at the corpse in front of him. "And now, he's dead."

Terrel nodded. "I'm wondering if he saw something that could lead us to the murderer. We wired him before we released him. He overheard an SUEC guard reporting an incident in which Ingrid Maulvi spiked a party drink. And he talked briefly with Dr. Robinson about the repair of an antenna."

"Did I hear my name?" Dr. Robinson appeared behind them. His stylish appearance and broad smile were flawless, as usual, as if he had just stepped out of a designer magazine.

He extended his hand to Angus. "Agent Weber, I'm so glad you are here now." He pointed at the corpse. "This is horrific. I hope you will resolve this case as quickly as possible."

Angus looked at him. "Agent Wright and I will do our best, Dr. Robinson."

Dr. Robinson nodded. "I am glad to hear that. Do you think Mr. Bezdomny killed himself? Perhaps he felt remorse. The gun that killed the student was found in his office. He was arrested earlier today. I wonder why he was released." He turned towards Terrel with a hostile gaze. "Do you have an explanation for that, Agent Wright?"

Terrel slowly removed the gloves from his hands. "Mr. Bezdomny was released because the gun in his office did not belong to him," he responded calmly.

"To whom *did* it belong?" Dr. Robinson asked.

"To one of the SUEC security guards. But the guard has an alibi for the time of Nia's death."

Dr. Robinson looked from Terrel to Angus. "So, Mr. Bezdomny stole the gun and shot Nia?"

"No. We have evidence that he was framed," Terrel responded.

"Who do you think framed him?" Oliver asked.

"We don't know that yet."

Oliver sighed and looked at Angus. "As I said, your team is completely in the dark. The reputation of our university and billions of donation dollars are at risk here. And I have to deal with amateurs."

Terrel took a deep breath. Another white guy who felt entitled to put him down.

Angus got up slowly. He was a few inches taller than the professor. He stepped towards him and looked down at him. "Dr. Robinson, I don't have the energy to pretend to like you today. Agent Wright and I are investigating a threat to the national security of the United States here. We are authorized to arrest suspects. *Anyone* who was in the building when this man hit the pavement could be a person of interest. Do you understand?"

Oliver Stuart Robinson responded with a broad smile. "I'm so glad you came to solve this case, Agent Weber! The SUEC security team already held up everyone who exited the building after the incident." He pointed at the two women in front of the building, who were looking at them from a distance. "I hope you will do your due diligence."

"Step aside, please." Two paramedics arrived with a stretcher, followed by an aftermath team.

"Let's give them some space." Angus stepped towards the research building. Then, turning to Dr. Robinson, he said, "I am afraid, you cannot be present when we interview anyone here. You are dismissed for now, but I would appreciate it if you would stay on the premises so that we can reach you if needed."

"Okay, I will wait in my office. Please debrief me after you've interviewed the suspects."

"You live on campus, right? You can go home if you like. We will contact you if we have any further questions for you. Our investigation is classified, and I doubt that I will have an update tonight."

"I'll stick around, just in case. You can find me in my office."

"It's your decision if you want to wait in your office. Just stay clear of the stairs to the roof and the roof area. They have been sealed."

"Thank you for your service, Agent Weber!"

Terrel felt the sting of being completely ignored. Angus looked at him from the corner of his eye. He put his arm around Terrel's shoulders and led him away with a gentle push. "Don't let him get under your skin, Terrel," he whispered as they walked away. "He's not worth it."

"He was also in the building when the man fell off the roof," Terrel exclaimed. "In fact, he was the last person who talked with him."

"I know. But that's not enough evidence for an arrest."

"Do you *really* think one of these women can throw a six-foot muscle head off the roof?" Terrel pointed at the two slim women, who were watching them as they approached.

"Never underestimate the strength of a woman," Angus said with a grin. "Let's just see if they had a chance and a motive."

The SUEC guard beside the two women greeted them eagerly. "It is such an honor to meet you, Agent Weber! I've heard so much about you!"

"Thank you! Actually, my colleague, Agent Wright, is leading this investigation." Angus pointed at Terrel. "I just came to assist."

"Of course. Hello, Agent Wright. Great to meet you as well."

Terrel nodded. "Thank you for waiting for us."

The guard pointed at the two women. "This is Dr. Lili Pham, radiologist at SUEC, and this is Dr. Aleshanee Dosela, who cleans the building every evening between 7 and 8 PM."

"A doctor who cleans the building?"

The young woman nodded. "I am a postdoctoral fellow here, and I'm earning extra money by cleaning the building in the evenings."

Terrel looked at her with raised eyebrows. "Really? Does the university not pay you enough?"

She shrugged. "The Bay Area is expensive. My sister is a student here as well, and we both live from my income."

Terrel looked at her again. She was tall and thin, with delicate facial features and kajal-outlined dark brown eyes. *Beautiful.* And poor. A second-class citizen in a first-class world. How did it feel to be a poor student at the wealthiest University in the world?

"Wow, it's impressive that you support both yourself and your sister," he said.

She looked at her hands. "I didn't really have much of a choice," she said coolly.

"Your family must be very proud of you," Angus added.

"Well, they are, and they aren't. They don't really understand what a postdoc is. All they understand is that the payment is bad. They wait for the big return from all those years of studying and missing family gatherings."

"I am sure it will come eventually," Terrel said softly.

"I hope it does," the woman said.

"Did you notice anything unusual tonight?" Terrel asked.

"Apart from the man who fell from the roof? No. I came here at 7 PM, as usual. We have robots that clean the floors and washrooms, you know. I only have to clean the trash cans in the research labs, collect any trash that people leave elsewhere, and dust off the art pieces in the building. I started with the offices on the upper floors and then worked my way down. I saw the building manager walking up the stairs, but I didn't think much of it."

"Why can the robot not clean the trash cans?"

"SUEC researchers are training robots for that, but apparently, the robots are not ready for that yet—there are too many containers in the lab that could be mistaken for a trash can. Some time ago, a robot cleaned out a specimen bin in a research lab. And a robot cannot yet recognize random trash lying around somewhere. So, humans have to take care of that part."

"That's interesting. So, you have to enter every lab and every office in this building to do your job?"

"That is correct."

"Did you notice any unusual trash today?"

"Well, there were computer pieces in three different trash cans. I don't know if they were from one or several computers. But usually, one just discards an old computer as one piece. These pieces were smashed. They looked like a bulldozer had run over them."

Terrel made a note. "That's interesting. Anything else?"

"Someone had thrown two green contact lenses in a white paper towel into a trash can on the first floor. When I first looked at it, I thought two eyeballs were looking at me. It completely spooked me!"

Terrel's jaw dropped. "You mean contact lenses with green irises?"

"That's correct, sir."

Terrel took a deep breath. This whole time, he had focused on a suspect with green eyes, and it was probably just a diversion. The killer had used green contact lenses. And they'd discarded them in this building.

"What is it, Terrel?" Lili asked.

"Well, we had been searching for a suspect with green eyes. Looks like it was a diversion."

Lili smiled. "In the radiology world, we call that *satisfaction of search*. You get hung up on a specific finding, and you miss another finding that is right in front of you."

"What does that have to do with anything?" Dr. Dosela asked.

"Well, in this case, the detectives might have focused on suspects with green eyes and not seen the obvious suspect right in front of them."

"Fascinating!" she said.

"Well, we will certainly set this straight," Terrel said, then turned to Dr. Dosela. "Where did you discard the trash?"

"In the container behind the building," she responded.

Terrel pulled his cell phone and asked the SUEC security team to secure the contents of the trash container. "Who did you see in the building today?" he asked.

Dr. Dosela thought for a moment. "Two students left shortly after I arrived," she said. "Dr. Diaz was in her office, and Dr. Robinson was in his lab on the second floor."

"Did you see anyone else walking up the stairs?"

"No, I didn't see anyone."

"Did you hear anything unusual?"

"No. But I had my headphones on. I only realized what had happened when I stepped out of the building."

Terrel looked at the young woman, processing the information "Did you see this woman today?" he asked her, pointing at Lili.

Dr. Dosela nodded. "Yes, I did. She was working on her computer when I came into her office shortly before 8 PM. It is on the first floor, one of my last stations. She told me that I didn't have to clean it today, which was great. I then continued cleaning the foyer."

"And you didn't see Dr. Pham walking up the stairs while you were cleaning the lobby?"

"No, I did not."

"Is there any other way to get to the roof?"

"One could take the elevator, but it's also in the foyer. I would have seen her. Then, of course, someone could have climbed the building from the outside. You know, like James Bond."

Terrel smiled at Lili. "I guess you have an alibi, Lili."

Lili exhaled sharply. "I'm glad to hear that."

"Did *you* notice anything that could help us find out what happened?" Terrel asked.

Lili shook her head. "Not late this evening, no, but earlier this afternoon, I believe I saw Ingrid walking up the stairs. She wore a hoodie, so there's a slight chance that I mixed her up with somebody. But I believe it was her. It's peculiar, because I heard from my colleagues that she had been kidnapped and escaped, so I wondered if she stopped by the research building before or after she was kidnapped. And why?"

"Did you talk with her?"

"No, I didn't. I only saw her from a distance."

"Thanks, that's interesting indeed. I'll check this out."

Lili got up from her bench. "I'm exhausted. I would really like to go."

"I'm so sorry we've kept you waiting," Terrel said. "You look really tired. Make sure to get some sleep."

Lili nodded. "As soon as I get a chance, I will."

A white man in a gray suit came down the path with long strides. Dean Hill greeted the group from a distance. "Hello, Agent Wright and Agent Weber! Hello, Dr. Pham! Hello, Mrs.?"

"Dr. Dosela."

"Oh, my apologies—another doctor! Under other circumstances, I would say it's a pleasure to meet you." He looked at the FBI agents. "I heard of the death of the building manager and came right away. Do you think it was an accident?"

Angus turned to the two women. "Thank you very much, doctors. You can go now."

Dr. Dosela got up and walked down the path towards the street, and Lili turned around and walked back to the research building. "Where are you going, Lili?" Terrel asked.

"I'll take a nap in my office," she said. "I live in San Francisco, and I don't feel alert enough to drive down the highway right now."

Terrel pointed at the octagon. "A man was probably murdered in that building."

Lili shrugged. "Well, if anyone wanted to kill me, they probably would've done it already. I was in the building all evening. I'm just too tired to drive right now. Right now, there's a higher chance that I will die in a car accident than from a gunshot. I don't want to end up like Nia."

Terrel nodded. "That's certainly your decision. You have my number. Call or text me if you see anything unusual."

He watched her as she disappeared into the building. He had a bad feeling knowing that both she and Dr. Robinson were in the building. They didn't get along, and it was not clear if somebody else was still in the building, hiding from the SUEC search team—the person who had pushed the manager from the roof. An SUEC security guard was blocking the stairs to the roof, but other accidents could happen. Should he ask Lili to stay here, on the front porch, where he could keep an eye on her and make sure she was safe? But she had looked really tired. The killer had likely fled the scene, and if they were still hiding somewhere, they would not have the audacity to attack another SUEC team member right in front of the FBI.

Angus Weber and Dean Hill had updated each other while Terrel spoke with the two women. He turned back to them now.

"Two witnesses heard Jacub cry as he fell off the building and said that it did not sound like a voluntary jump," he explained. "In addition, I talked with the victim shortly before his death, and there was no indication whatsoever of suicidal plans. He agreed to be tape wired. I can't imagine that someone would do that if they were planning to jump off a building."

"He was tape-wired? Did you record anything that revealed that he was pushed of the roof?" Dean Hill asked.

"We're working on that," Terrel responded. "There might have been the footsteps of a second person on the roof shortly before his death, but it's not enough to identify anyone."

"So, you still have no leads?" Dean Hill asked.

"Well, Lili—Dr. Pham—reported that she saw a man with a gun in the park earlier today, after the alleged attack on Dr. Maulvi."

"So, there was a shooter after all?"

"Well, yes and no. Lili took a picture with her iPhone, and it was Nia's father. I had met him earlier this morning, and I recognized him."

"So, he may be on a mission to avenge his daughter?"

"I am afraid that might be the case. He is a licensed concealed gun carrier. I cannot arrest him for simply carrying a gun in his pocket, but I did alert the SUEC security team and the local police. They have an eye on him. Be wary if you encounter him."

"Of course. I feel sorry for him. No parent should have to bury their own child. He must be going through immense emotional turmoil."

"Agree. Just be careful. Desperate parents are unpredictable."

"Where is Mr. Johnes now?" Angus Weber asked.

"Let me check with my team." Terrel typed something into his phone. It buzzed a few minutes later—a text message. Terrel looked at the screen and then at Angus.

"What is it?" he asked.

Terrel read the message. "Mr. Johnes among the spectators in front of the research building. Lost contact. Disappeared in the park."

Dean Hill threw both hands in the air. "Oh, my god. He was here the whole time? Did *he* push the manager of the roof? The murder weapon was found in Jacub's office earlier today, right? Did Mr. Johnes hear that and take revenge?"

"Let's not jump to conclusions," Angus responded. "He was among the spectators. We do not know if he was in the building."

"I will find him," Terrel said. He turned around and walked down the gravel path into the park.

- 35 -

ANNYA

The Tip
Wednesday, May 25, 2033, 9:00 p.m.

Annya went to the nurse station in the ER, where several nurses were working on computers. It had been relatively calm here half an hour ago, but now, it was busy. Ridiculously busy.

Annya peeked around the corner towards the reception area. People of every gender and shape were moving around. Physicians, nurses and technicians were hurrying in and out of the exam rooms The waiting room and hallways were filled with patients. A child was crying in the distance. A nurse calling for an x-ray technician. A resident physician rushing for the crash cart.

This was the ER in action. Everyone worked until they were exhausted, thirsty, hungry, and desperate to go home. And yet, most came back the next day, determined to do the right things.

A nurse came out of the trauma care room, blood spattered over her white coat and face. "Hi, Lidia. Do you need help?" Annya asked.

"No, we're fine," the nurse said with a hoarse voice. "Gunshot victim. On his way to the OR."

Annya nodded.

"We didn't have a doc to look at the patient next door," the nurse said, pointing at another exam room. "An elderly lady with abdominal pain."

"Take a break. I'll have a look," Annya said.

"Thank you!"

Annya looked at the medical file in front of the door. Violine Johnes. Johnes with an h. Was this a coincidence?

Annya knocked at the door. Nobody answered. She opened the door and asked, "Can I come in?"

An elderly black lady was sitting on a stretcher, holding her belly with her left hand. "Of course," she said.

"Hi, I am Dr. Annya Segond, ER physician here."

The lady extended her hand. "I am Violine Johnes. Nice to meet you."

Annya looked at her. Perhaps there was some resemblance. "Do you happen to be related to Nia Johnes?" she asked.

"Yes, I'm her mother. Or was." Tears glinted in her eyes. She blinked them away.

"My sincere condolences. She will always be your daughter."

"Did you know her?"

"A little."

"Did you treat her for her pneumonia? She was treated here, wasn't she?"

"Yes, I did see her when she came in for the first time. She was very sick and waited for almost two hours in the waiting room. When it was her turn, she asked that the man next to her be seen first. He had a bad forearm fracture and was in severe pain. It is very rare that people do that in the ER. Most think only of themselves."

"Yes, this was her. Always watching out for others."

"And now you came here with belly pain?"

"Yes, we had fried calamari for lunch today. I love the seafood here. But my stomach does not tolerate fried food. I just needed it for comfort today. And then, this evening, I had to face the consequences. I suddenly felt a sharp pain under my ribcage, here, that extended into my shoulder." She pointed at her right upper abdomen and right shoulder.

"Hm, can I have a look?" Annya washed her hands at the sink and walked over to Mrs. Johnes. She palpated her right upper abdomen.

"Ouch!" the woman exclaimed.

Annya looked at the information on the computer. Mrs. Johnes had a fever. The ultrasound technician had attempted an ultrasound, but it was difficult to interpret due to Mrs. Johnes's body habitus. She had been sent for a quick MRI scan, a new service here in the ER. Annya looked at the scan. It showed a large stone in the gallbladder and a markedly enhancing gallbladder wall.

"You have a large stone in your gallbladder and inflammation," Annya explained.

The woman sighed. "I know that I have gallbladder stones. They act up whenever I am stressed."

"Fortunately, the stones did not get stuck anywhere and did not cause any obstruction. I'll prescribe some antibiotics for you," Annya said. "You should feel better very soon."

"I hope so," the woman said.

It was silent for a while. Annya entered information into Mrs. Johnes's file on the computer, and Mrs. Johnes closed her eyes. "I wish I could talk with her just one more time," she said after a while. "Every now and then, I see something that reminds me of her, and then I feel this deep pain again. I miss her so much."

Annya had completed her entries and was ready to leave. She wasn't particularly good at comforting grieving parents. She would get the counselor here. She just needed to find the right moment to say goodbye. "You must have been very proud that Nia went to SUEC."

"Indeed, I was at the time, but now, I wish she had never gone to this godforsaken place."

"I understand."

"It's all my fault. When my husband and I had just married, he was diagnosed with cancer. After he completed his chemotherapy, he could not conceive a child for a while, so we decided to conceive a child with a sperm donor."

"That sounds like a good solution, under the circumstances."

"Well, I wanted to choose the smartest donor available. And that was a professor. He happened to be white. I wanted our child to be smart—to have opportunities, you know."

Annya looked at the woman. She didn't know what to say.

"I would have taken a black professor if they had one. But black professors don't donate sperm. Do you know why that is?"

"I'm afraid I don't."

"Well, I thought it was a trivial detail. But my husband just found out, and he is really mad."

"Perhaps you can assure him that this does not change his relationship with his daughter. He was the one who raised her."

"You don't understand. He just found out that Dr. Stuart Robinson is Nia's biological father. Nia found out that he was involved in illegal business at SUEC, and she was killed here!"

Annya looked at the woman, processing the information. "Illegal business?"

The woman nodded. "He played with people's genes, if I understood correctly."

"And where is your husband now? He didn't come with you?"

"He stormed out of our apartment. I don't know where he went. He has a gun. I'm really concerned. I wanted to follow him, but first, I had to deal with the dog."

"A dog?" Annya could not believe her ears. There were not that many dogs on campus.

The woman nodded. "A German Shepherd. He followed us on the street, and we took him in. Such a sweet boy. And you know, the funny thing is, he had a memory stick on his collar with Nia's birth certificate on it. Can you imagine that? It was like a miracle."

"A memory stick?"

"Yes, a memory stick with information about illegal business here at SUEC. The dog had it on his collar."

"And the dog did what?"

"My husband slammed the door in his face, and he started to bark. I tried to calm him down, but couldn't. So, I just opened the door, and he ran after my husband. I wanted to follow them, but then I got this excruciating pain. I couldn't move. I tried, but it only got worse. I sat down on the sidewalk and nearly fainted. A student found me there and called an ambulance. That's how I got here."

"And your husband went where?"

"I don't know. Perhaps he is looking for the professor. I'm so scared that he might do something stupid. He is the only one I've got left." A stream of tears rolled down her face.

"If he is on the SUEC campus, we'll find him," Annya said. "I will inform our security team, and they'll look for him."

"He's a good man. Nia's death is just too much for him."

"We'll find him. Excuse me for a minute."

Annya went to the nursing station and provided instructions for Mrs. Johnes's care. Then, she grabbed her jacket and left the ER. It would be best to check things out by herself. She would call Terrel from the airplane.

She walked over to the landing pad for electric vertical take-off and landing aircrafts (eVTOL), a large evenly cemented circle to the right of the hospital. An SUEC eVTOL shuttle had just taken off. The white painted aircraft looked like a small helicopter with four radiating wings and power propellors. The electric motor produced very little noise, like a gust of wind. One of the passengers looked at Annya through the window. Was that Ingrid Maulvi?

Annya put her hand over her eyes to see better. It was dark outside, and the ambient light in the aircraft barely illuminated the faces of the passengers, but after looking carefully, she was sure: it was Ingrid indeed! She must have left her hospital room. There was a guard at the door, but perhaps she had escaped through the window. What was she thinking? She needed intravenous antibiotics. Otherwise, her osteomyelitis would become much worse very quickly.

The next eVTOL shuttle arrived on the landing pad. Annya waited for the passengers to disembark. Then, she took a seat, and a few minutes later, she was on her way to the SUEC campus as well. A full moon illuminated the beautiful scenery below her—lights from streetlamps and houses in Redwood city, a chain of cars driving down the US-101 highway, the San Francisco Bay in the distance, gentle hills with emerald-green Redwood trees that swayed in the evening breeze.

Her phone rang. It was Charles, the chief technician from the genetics lab. "Hi, Annya. We got initial results from the sperm samples that you sent to us. I have to run a few more tests for confirmation, but it looks like all the samples have a *CCR5*-delta32 homozygous genotype."

"Wow. That is the same gene that the biophysicist He Jiankui edited a few years ago, right? He created the CRISPR babies that were supposed to be resistant to HIV infections?"

"Exactly! But, in this case, I did not find any evidence for genetic editing. I believe these are natural samples. They have just been selected based on the presence of this mutation."

"That is exactly what we expected. Thanks so much, Charles. This was extremely helpful. Can you please prepare a written summary? I will pick it up tomorrow."

"Of course."

The eVTOL shuttle had reached the landing pad at SUEC University. Annya got out and dialed Terrel's phone number.

"Hello, this is Agent Wright."

"Hi, Terrel. I just saw Mrs. Johnes in the hospital—Nia's mother. Mr. Johnes is on campus with a gun. Check on him."

"Thanks for letting me know. I'm already on it."

"The German Shepherd was at his apartment. The Johneses found a chip with evidence on his collar."

"I'll send somebody to retrieve it."

"Thanks. Be careful."

"You too. See you at the research building?"

"Yes, I just landed at the SUEC eVTOL landing base. I'll come over now."

"Great. Angus Weber is there as well. See you soon."

Annya hung up the phone. Her heart jumped a little. These were unfortunate circumstances, but she was looking forward to seeing the FBI director again.

She did not notice the shadow watching her from behind the rhododendron bushes.

***

Ingrid waited until Annya had left. Then, she took off in the opposite direction. In front of her was the SUEC golf course. Several golf carts were parked to her right. *How convenient.*

Ingrid jumped in and drove toward the SUEC valley.

- 36 -

SCHNITZEL

The Reunion
Wednesday, May 25, 2033, 9:30 p.m.

Schnitzel ran down the street, trying to find the scent of the angry man. What was he thinking, storming out of the apartment like that? Did he not know that the coyotes would come back, looking for revenge? They would feel emboldened by the darkness of the night. And by finding the old man alone.

Schnitzel had to rescue this stupid human.

He put his snout into the air. Above him was a dark night sky with millions of sparkling stars. An owl passed by. He growled, and it disappeared into the nearby park. His sensitive muzzle detected a faint fragrance to his right—the old man.

Schnitzel followed it. It was the same path via which they had come here. Was the scent that he smelled from a few hours ago? No, it was not lingering on the bushes along his path. It was hanging in the air. Schnitzel was quite sure it was fresh. The man was walking back to the place where they had found the dead man.

What did he not understand about avoiding human killers? They were much worse than the coyotes.

Schnitzel ran faster. An alley of solar trees on each side of the university street gently illuminated his path. The scent became stronger. He was getting closer.

Schnitzel saw a moving figure in the distance. That was the man. He was walking towards the research building at the end of the street. A small breeze was blowing towards Schnitzel, carrying a confusing scent of many different humans, mingled with human blood. *Scary.*

In the distance, the moving shadow of the old man merged with multiple others in front of the research building. Another gentle breeze rolled towards Schnitzel, carrying another potpourri of human scents to him. But there was something else—another scent. It was faint, but breathtakingly familiar.

Schnitzel stopped to catch it in its entirety. No doubt—it was Heinz!

Schnitzel howled as loud as he could, then raced toward a cloud of humans in front of the research building. They all looked in the same direction, towards the research building, not paying any attention to him.

Except one.

"Schnitzel?" he heard Heinz's voice ask.

Schnitzel barked in agreement. *Yes, it's me. Where are you? It's me. I missed you so much. Where are you?*

A huge young man disentangled from the human congregation and slowly walked towards the large dog who was racing towards him. Heinz recognized him as well. He fell to his knees, arms wide open. "Schnitzel!" he exclaimed.

Schnitzel barked again. *Yes, it's me. I'm so glad I found you!* He jumped into Heinz's arms, toppling him over and licking his face.

Heinz laughed and embraced his beloved dog. "I am so glad I found you!" he said softly. Schnitzel jumped up and down, wagging his tail, snuggling his human life-partner, rolling around and exposing his belly for rubs. Heinz happily engaged, laughing uncontrollably, forgetting everything around him.

Several of the other humans turned around to watch the spectacle. "Did you lose your dog?" someone asked.

"Yes, he was kidnapped!" Heinz exclaimed breathlessly. "I didn't know if he was alive or if I would ever see him again. I'm so happy I found him!"

"Good for you," the man responded, turning back to the scene at the research building. So did the other humans.

Schnitzel recognized another familiar smell. He lifted his head. The angry old man was standing just a few meters away, looking at him through the crowd. Schnitzel wanted to jump at him, but Heinz held him back by his collar. "Hey, my friend, you don't want to run away again?"

Heinz ruffled Schnitzel's head and scratched him behind his ears. Schnitzel loved that. He licked Heinz's face, and Heinz laughed again.

He produced a treat from his pocket. Schnitzel happily accepted. That was his Heinz!

He looked back at the area where the old man had been standing. He was gone.

Heinz started to examine Schnitzel's collar. His brows furrowed. *Why are humans so emotionally unstable?* Schnitzel felt his heart sink. *This is exhausting. Can Heinz not stay happy for more than a few minutes?*

Heinz had pulled off the small cap of the memory stick, but the main part was gone. Heinz held the cap in front of Schnitzel's nose. "Schnitzel, you were supposed to guard this," he said in a serious tone.

Schnitzel looked at Heinz, head tilted. *What does he want?*

"Schnitzel, where is the rest of this memory stick?" Heinz demanded, holding the cap again in front of him. "Find it!"

Schnitzel barked. He knew what Heinz wanted! He would lead him to the memory stick, and then Heinz would surely reward him with another treat.

Schnitzel turned around and ran back down the street to where he had come from. "Schnitzel, wait!" Heinz came running after him. Schnitzel waited for his owner to catch up. When Heinz came into arm-length distance, Schnitzel ran forward again.

And so on until they had reached the apartment building.

- 37 -

HEINZ

The Attack
Wednesday, May 25, 2033, 10:00 p.m.

Heinz Tremblay followed Schnitzel down the road to a large apartment building. They walked through the entrance, up the stairs and down a long white-painted hallway.

Schnitzel sat down in front of an apartment door at the end of the hallway, looking at the door. Heinz searched for a bell. There was none. He knocked.

No response.

He knocked again.

No response.

He knocked again, and the door gave in a little. Heinz pushed. It was not completely closed. He could push it open.

"Hello?" he called into the entrance area.

Silence.

Schnitzel squeezed himself through the space between the doorframe and Heinz's legs, disappearing into an adjacent room. Heinz followed. Schnitzel sat upright in the kitchen, looking at Heinz and then at a loaf of bread on the counter. Heinz shook his head. "Schnitzel, all you can think of is food."

Schnitzel's tail wagged up and down on the kitchen floor.

Heinz shook his head. He walked into the adjacent living room. "Hello?" he asked again. Schnitzel followed reluctantly. There was nobody in the living room, either.

A laptop was on a coffee table beside the sofa. Heinz stepped closer. His memory stick was in it!

"Well done!" He patted Schnitzel's head. The dog looked back at him with pride and walked back into the kitchen. Heinz got what he wanted. And Schnitzel had made clear what *he* wanted.

Heinz smiled. He was so happy that he'd found his beloved dog again, but he had to check first that they were safe here. He continued to walk through the apartment. He found a bedroom with a neatly made bed with white blankets and light-green velvet throw pillows. Adjacent was a small bathroom. There was nobody here.

Heinz went back into the kitchen. Schnitzel did deserve a little treat. The dog sat upright in front of the counter, staring at the bread.

Heinz broke off a generous piece. The owners would hopefully not mind. He would pay them when they came back. Schnitzel grunted in approval. Heinz handed the bread to him, and Schnitzel swallowed it in one piece. He licked his lips as if to say, "More please!"

Heinz looked around. There was a bowl on the floor. *Did the people who lived in the apartment also have a dog? Or did they feed Schnitzel? Then they couldn't be that bad.* Heinz took a glass, got water from the sink, and filled the bowl. Schnitzel drank.

Heinz went back into the living room. There were photos on the coffee table beside the couch. He recognized the face immediately.

It was Nia.

He sat down on the couch and looked through them. Nia as a child. Nia in front of the SUEC entrance, laughing into the camera. Nia in the lab, holding an Eppendorf tube, smiling. Nia with an elderly couple. Her parents?

Below the photos was a letter from the Dean informing Mr. and Mrs. Johnes about the tragic passing of their daughter. Heinz looked around. This had to be the apartment where Nia's parents were staying. They had likely received Nia's belongings.

And Schnitzel might have picked up the scent.

Heinz looked at the laptop on the ottoman in front of him. A USB drive was sticking out of its right side. He grabbed it. He had to check if the data on the memory stick had been accessed from the thumb drive or downloaded onto the computer hard drive. Schnitzel came in and settled on the carpet, leaning against him.

Heinz tried to open the computer. A window appeared on the screen, asking for a username and password. Heinz tried a few options. No luck. Perhaps he should just take both the laptop and the memory stick.

Nia had been killed, he had been drugged, and Schnitzel had been kidnapped because of what was on that thumb drive. It could be dangerous here. Perhaps they should leave.

Schnitzel jumped up and growled. Heinz looked up. Were there footsteps in the hallway? Yes, there was someone coming down the hallway. *Tap. Tap. Tap.*

There was a shuffling noise in front of the door. Heinz felt beads of sweat running down his temples. The door squeaked.

He got up from the couch and looked around. There was a silver candelabra on the shelf besides the fireplace. He grabbed it. Schnitzel jumped up and started barking uncontrollably. Heinz snatched his collar to hold him back. He didn't want the dog to bite the owner of the apartment, and he felt safer with the dog close to him.

The steps came closer. Now, they were in the foyer. Then, the outline of a women appeared in the door frame.

"Ingrid!" Heinz exclaimed. "What are *you* doing here?"

Ingrid stared at him in surprise. "Hello, Heinz. I could ask you the same thing."

Heinz placed the candelabra back on the shelf. "Well, Schnitzel brought me here. I don't know why. He somehow knew this place. Based on the photos I found here, I'm assuming that Nia's parents are staying here." He pointed at the photos and letter in front of him.

Ingrid nodded. "Perhaps Schnitzel picked up Nia's scent here."

Schnitzel continued to bark at her. "What are *you* doing here?" Heinz asked again.

"I was discharged from the hospital and didn't want to go home. I thought I'd go meet Nia's parent's and express my condolences. I was told that they were supposed to be staying here."

Heinz nodded. "I'm afraid they're not here." He pulled the dog by his collar. "Shush! It's just Ingrid." Schnitzel continued to bark at her.

Ingrid looked at him. "He still doesn't like me. I don't understand why." She stepped closer. Schnitzel jumped forward and snapped at her.

"Stop it!" Heinz exclaimed. "I'm really sorry, Ingrid. I don't know what got into him. He was perfectly calm just a minute ago."

"Never mind," she said. "We all had a hard day today."

"You're right," Heinz responded. "But that does not justify getting aggressive. I'll let him cool off."

He dragged Schnitzel to the kitchen, pushed him in, and closed the door. Schnitzel jumped at the door from the other side, barking frantically.

Heinz turned back to Ingrid. "How are *you* feeling? " He pointed at the bandage on her hand.

"I'm doing okay," she said. "It still hurts, but I believe the wounds are healing. I just feel a little weak." She walked to the couch and sat down.

Heinz joined her. He leaned forward and pulled the memory stick out of the computer.

"Is this your computer?" Ingrid asked with an innocent smile.

Heinz got a funny feeling. Perhaps it was better to keep the memory stick to himself. Nia could have easily handed it over to Ingrid in the lab next door—but she didn't.

"No, the computer was here already," Heinz responded. "The memory stick is mine. I wanted to meet Nia's parents as well. I wanted to wait for them and work on the computer in the meantime. But, of course, I don't know the password to login."

Ingrid smiled. "You're always working." She got up and walked over to the balcony door. The apartment was on the second floor, built on a hillside. The living room had a large sliding glass door that led to a small balcony. Ingrid opened the doors and stepped out. "It's a beautiful summer night out here," she said.

Heinz didn't know what to say. Schnitzel was still barking in the kitchen. He felt guilty for leaving him there. They had just found each other again, but he could not risk him biting Ingrid.

Ingrid stood outside. Her silky long hair was blown backwards by a summer breeze. Her face was so smooth and flawless, like a porcelain doll. Heinz looked at her. The full moon softened her outline. She was so beautiful.

He walked over to her. A cool evening breeze embraced them. "What is that?" she asked, pointing at the memory stick in his hand.

"Nothing special," he said. "Just work."

"Can I see it?"

That was a little weird. What did she want with a memory stick here? She wouldn't be able to read it. "Sure." Heinz handed it to her.

She smiled at him, embraced by a million stars on the navy-blue sky. He had always wondered how it would feel to kiss her. She came closer. "I'm really glad you came," he said softly.

"I didn't expect to find you here. What a coincidence," she whispered. Their lips were only a few micrometers apart.

There was a metallic sound on the balcony floor. "Oopsy," Ingrid said. She stepped forward and stomped on the memory stick.

"Oh, no!" Heinz exclaimed.

Ingrid lifted her foot and stomped on it again with force. It burst.

Heinz stared at her. "Did you do that on purpose?" he exclaimed in disbelief. "Why would you do that?"

Ingrid kicked the broken pieces through the railing of the balcony into an adjacent rose bush. "I'm sorry, Heinz," she said in a soothing voice. Then, in a split second, her arm shot up, and she grabbed his throat.

"What are you doing?" he managed to say, gasping for air. Ingrid was half his size in all dimensions. Was she going to harm him? He tried to push her away, but she somehow stood her ground. Her grip around his neck tightened.

He felt dizzy. He tried to grab her arms. But she pushed him backwards, over the railing. Heinz reached for the railing to avoid falling backwards.

"You're hurting me," he managed to say before the world around him started spinning. Ingrid's contours became blurry and started to fade. He could not breathe. His hands on the railing went limp.

Schnitzel barked frantically, scratching at the kitchen door.

Suddenly, two sharp thudding sounds filled the air. Heinz felt as if an angry bee had just passed by. Gunshots!

Ingrid let out a cry and released her grip on Heinz's throat. She clutched her right shoulder. Heinz gasped for air.

"Don't move. I have a gun!" A woman approached them from the living room, her arms extended, holding a gun.

Heinz stared at the gun barrel pointing at him. Or Ingrid? He wasn't sure.

"Oh, Annya, thank you so much for coming to my rescue!" Ingrid exclaimed. "Heinz wanted to assault me! I found out that *he* was the one who kidnapped me earlier today. And he tried it again."

Heinz stared at her in disbelief. He opened his mouth to speak, but words wouldn't come out. His neck was swollen. It was hard to breathe. He coughed profusely.

"Is that so?" Annya responded coldly. "Why was your hand around his throat, then? It seems that *he* is injured."

"He attacked me. I was defending myself."

"I would never harm anyone," Heinz managed to say with a creaky voice. "Ingrid destroyed my memory stick."

Ingrid scoffed. "What memory stick? Do you see one anywhere here?" She held her bandaged hand in the air and glared at Heinz. "Your dog attacked me, and *you* wanted to hurt me. You are a bad liar, Heinz!"

Heinz looked at her in disbelief. Everyone he met was just using him. And hurting him. He was deeply disappointed. "I thought you were my friend," he murmured.

"You will both come with me," Annya said calmly. "You can tell your story to the FBI, and they'll check the evidence. You do not invent the truth. Facts create the truth."

"Thank you!" Heinz said. "I would be happy to talk with the FBI." He stepped towards Annya. She looked alarmed.

He realized too late that his body had intersected the line between her and Ingrid.

Ingrid seized the moment. She grabbed the railing with her bandaged hand and jumped over it.

"Stop!" Annya leaped forward, reaching for her. But she only reached into the air. The darkness of the night was on Ingrid's side. She hit the ground on the other side and quickly limped into the adjacent park.

Annya sent several gun shots after her, but her silhouette became blurry, and she disappeared behind the opulent rhododendron bushes.

"Drop your weapon!" a voice behind them shouted. Heinz saw an SUEC guard entering the living room, aiming at Annya. She turned around slowly.

"Drop your weapon, or I will shoot you!" the guard said again.

Annya dropped the gun and put her arms up. "I am Dr. Annya Segond, CIA," she said calmly.

"Don't shoot her. She saved my life!" Heinz added.

"Where is your ID?" the guard asked.

"In my right pocket," Annya responded.

The guard came closer, reached into her pocket, and produced the CIA badge. He looked at her with suspicion, but then put his gun down. "Who is he?" He pointed at Heinz.

"A victim. It seems that he had sensitive information on a memory stick, which was destroyed. The person of interest is Dr. Ingrid Maulvi. She just jumped off the balcony here. We need to find her."

The guard stepped back and dialed a number on his phone.

Schnitzel was still barking frantically in the kitchen. "Can I check on my dog?" Heinz asked.

The guard nodded. "If you keep him in check. If he threatens me, I will shoot him."

"I will make sure he doesn't bother you." Heinz opened the kitchen door, and Schnitzel jumped out, barking at everyone. Heinz held his dog close, trying to calm him down.

The guard stepped back into the foyer, talking on the phone. Schnitzel continued to bark frantically. Heinz knelt down and embraced him. Schnitzel leaned into him but showed his teeth and growled at Annya.

Annya stood still and turned to the side with her head down. Schnitzel looked at her with a tilted head. Did he recognize her? Annya slightly turned away, keeping him in her peripheral vision. Then, she extended her hand to him. Schnitzel sniffed at her hand and then greeted her with a wagging tail. She patted his head.

The guard returned. Schnitzel growled again, fletching his teeth. "Schnitzel, stop it!" Heinz said in a stern voice.

"I just talked with Professor Robinson," the guard said. "There must be a misunderstanding. Dr. Ingrid Maulvi is one of his employees. He said that she was never violent and has no criminal record whatsoever. He asked me to bring you to the research building. The FBI is there, and they can check your story."

"Will you send somebody after Ingrid?" Annya asked.

"You said that she ran into the park. It is unlikely that we'll find her there in the dark. She could be anywhere by now. We'll wait until she reappears."

"She assaulted me!" Heinz exclaimed. "She might endanger somebody else."

The guard shrugged. "She ran into the park. How should I find her in the dark? You can discuss this with Agent Weber. He'll decide what to do."

Annya sighed. There was no point trying to reach this man. He had made up his mind already. Hopefully, Terrel and Angus would untangle this nonsense. "Okay, let's go," she said.

Heinz produced a leash from his jacket, put Schnitzel on it, and the four—three humans and a dog—left the premises.

- 38 -

ANNYA

The Revenge
Wednesday, May 25, 2033, 10:30 p.m.

Annya, Heinz, and Schnitzel arrived at the research building. The SUEC guard led Annya to the FBI agents.

"I found a woman with green eyes and a gun in Mr. and Mrs. Johnes's apartment," he said with satisfaction in his voice.

Terrel looked at Annya and shook his head. "She is one of us," he said. "And Mr. Tremblay is a victim, not a suspect. Please release them."

The guard looked disappointed but did as he was told. Annya held up her cuffed hands, rolling her eyes. "Sorry, Annya," Angus Weber said as the SUEC guard took the handcuffs off.

"No worries. I'm here now," she said. She briefed Angus, Terrel, and the Dean about the events at the apartment. Cristina had secured sperm samples from Dr. Robinson's lab that appeared to be enriched for the CCR5-delta32 gene, a gene that encoded resistance of the carrier to various infections. Heinz had found Nia's list of patients who had both a history of IVF and infections. The list stated that all of their infections resolved. Jacub had found PCR tests that showed that Nia, Ingrid and Heinz were conceived by the same sperm donor and carried the CCR5-delta32 gene. Their names were on the list.

"So, Nia found out that patients with the CCR5-delta32 gene recovered completely from various infections?" Angus summarized. "That is not a crime."

"The patients were all conceived by IVF, and this gene was likely selected for them without the mother's knowledge," Annya explained. "That is not allowed."

"But it is allowed to perform preimplantation diagnoses and discard embryos who carry genes that encode a disease?" Angus asked.

"Yes, that is correct," Annya explained. "IVF clinics nowadays test for many single-gene diseases such as Thalassemia, Duchenne muscular dystrophy, Huntington's disease, Cystic Fibrosis, certain Cancer Predisposition Syndromes, and several others. The goal here is to create health embryos. However, it is not allowed to select for random genes in healthy embryos, let alone to create designer babies by adding desired genes. This is because unintended changes can be passed down to children, grandchildren, and great-grandchildren. Any error, known or unknown, will affect future generations."

The Dean nodded. "If someone did that on a grand scale, they could rewrite the entire gene pool of future generations and change humanity as we know it."

"So, if Dr. Robinson created humans who carry a gene that makes them resistant to infections, how would he know that his creation worked? I mean, how would he know that these people were truly resistant to infections?" Heinz asked.

"It looks like Dr. Robinson and Dr. Maulvi created their own little experiment," Terrel explained. "We found out that Ingrid Maulvi deliberately infected people with bacteria or viruses without their knowledge or consent. Then they observed if the patient recovered from that infection. And they all did."

"Wow, that is incredible," Heinz said. "I remember how I recovered from my COVID-19 pneumonia. Perhaps it was good that I had this gene."

"Welcome to the era of preimplantation genetic testing and designer babies!" Annya said. "I am glad that you recovered from your infection. But there could be side effects that we do not understand yet. It is morally wrong to try to improve otherwise healthy embryos."

Suddenly, Schnitzel started to bark wildly. He jumped up and raced into the darkness behind the research building. "Schnitzel, stop!" Heinz exclaimed and took up the chase.

Angus and an SUEC guard ran after him. "Perhaps the dog smelled Ingrid. She is dangerous. Protect Annya and the Dean," Angus shouted back at Terrel.

"What is happening?" Dean Hill asked in an anxious voice.

Terrel pulled his gun. "No worries. I have you covered," he said, exploring the perimeter around them with a flashlight.

Angus and the guard disappeared behind the corner of the dimly lit octagonal limestone building. For a few moments, they did not hear or see anything.

Dean Hill's phone rang. He looked at the display, then took the call. "Hello, Atharv, how are you doing?" he said in a cheery voice. Annya looked at the Dean, who winked. "Yes, of course, I have thought about baby food. I'll stop at the grocery store on my way home and get some."

Annya could not hear the voice on the other end of the phone.

"Yes, I'm as excited as you are!" the Dean said. "Only two more days, and we'll be parents!"

They heard the dog howling horribly behind the building. Annya tried to see what was going on in the distance, but Angus and Heinz had been swallowed by the darkness of the night. She was not sure what to do. Protect the Dean or look after Angus and Heinz.

"No, honey, everything is fine here," the Dean said. "That must have been something on the radio. I'll turn it off."

There were some voices in the distance. They were coming back.

Dean Hill tried to keep his cheery tone. "Honey, I'm afraid I have to go. There's someone coming who needs to talk with me. See you soon!"

The Dean hung up, got a handkerchief from his pocket, and patted sweat beads on his forehead. Terrel looked at him. "Are you okay?"

The Dean nodded. "Sure. I just didn't want my husband to worry. He's so excited about our baby girl. I cannot ruin this. Please help me."

Annya looked from one man to the other. "I don't understand," she said.

The Dean turned towards her. "My husband and I are adopting a baby girl this weekend," he said. "Do you know where I can buy baby formula for a newborn?"

Annya shrugged. "Sorry, I don't have any children. And I believe we have more pressing problems on our hands right now."

"Walmart should do," Terrel said with a smirk.

"Thank you!" the Dean responded. "You're saving my life twice! I might escape the killer here, but if I return without the formula tonight, I will get killed at home!"

"Don't joke about this kind of thing," Terrel said with a serious look on his face.

A shadow parted from the darkness behind the research building and came towards them.

- 39 -

LILI

The Shadow
Wednesday, May 25, 2033, 10:30 p.m.

Lili had closed the door and crashed on the couch in her office. She was exhausted. The settee was short, but she curled up in it just fine, embraced by its tight back and arms. Her soft cape scarf aided as a snuggly blanket. The SUEC valley always cooled down in the evenings, when the nearby ocean sent cool winds inland.

Lili tightened the scarf around her and instantly fell into a deep, dreamless sleep—the sleep of the on-call physician attending. It restored some of her energy while preserving a certain amount of conscious awareness of her surroundings. The noise from ambulance sirens and people on the street outside had calmed down. Presumably, most of the spectators had left.

Distantly, Lili's sleeping mind noticed the evening wind rushing around the building, rustling the leaves of adjacent trees, and rattling the window frames. A raven croaked outside. It felt peaceful at last.

Lili's wandering mind mourned Nia's death. She remembered Nia's polite smile and attentive gaze when she'd met her in the research building—genuine, curious, a little guarded perhaps. Her musical, joyful laugh when she was chatting with her friends. She had been a beautiful, bright young woman, full of dreams for the future. Dead.

And Jacub. The most sincere, decent, well-mannered guy Lili had met at SUEC. An old-school gentleman, the kind of guy who always let a woman through the door first and held it for her. Perhaps a little rigid at first until they had gotten to know each other, and he'd turned out to be quite goofy. A friend you could count on. Dead.

It was hard to comprehend. Nia and Jacub, gone forever. What was left was Dr. Robinson's cruel smile.

Lili realized that it was not so much her body that needed rest. It was her *soul* that needed a break.

She wasn't sure how long she had been resting on the couch. A strange noise alerted her. Lili felt an adrenaline rush, as if someone had called her for an emergency. She sat up and checked her iPhone, but there was no call or text from the clinic.

There was a barking dog outside. Lili got up and walked to the window, which was facing the park along the right side of the research building. An array of blue LED lights dimly illuminated the perimeter of the research building.

A human shadow emerged from the park, walking towards the research building. It was too dark to tell who it was. Perhaps a woman. She had something in her hand. A big stick of some sort.

A large dog came racing towards the person, barking frantically. Lili held her breath. The person stood still for a moment, letting the dog approach. When it had almost reached her, the shadow lifted the stick. It glistened under the LED lights—a golf club!

The shadow hit the dog with full force. The dog cried out and fell to the ground, howling and whining. Lili gasped. Who would be so cruel as to hit a dog like that?

The shadow turned around and looked towards her. Lili felt a shiver running down her spine. She froze. The lights in her office were out. The woman could not possibly see her.

Then, she noted an SUEC guard coming around the corner, just underneath her window. The shadow was still mostly covered by the darkness of the park. The guard looked around, alerted by the howling dog, but he had not spotted the human yet. In a split-second, the shadow jumped forward and hit the guard in the head with the golf club. The guard cried out and fell to the ground, not moving. Was he dead?

The shadow jumped towards the guard, removed their SUEC cap and jacket, and put them on. Then, they patted the guard, produced a gun, and put it in their belt. The whole action had taken less than a minute.

They grabbed the lifeless guard and dragged him behind a dumpster at the back of the building. Then, the shadow disappeared towards the backside of the building.

Lili realized that she had held her breath all this time. She inhaled deeply.

But she did not get much time to think. Other voices were coming closer.

"Oh, my god, Schnitzel is injured!" a big man cried out, running towards the howling dog and kneeling beside him. "Help! He's bleeding!"

Two other men followed—an SUEC guard and a man with an FBI jacket. Not Terrel. Perhaps Agent Weber.

Lili stared at the three men. Should she say anything? But she hadn't made the best experiences with Agent Weber. The last time she'd met him, he had treated her as if she were the perpetrator. Who would believe her story that a woman came out of the woods, hit the dog, and disappeared?

"What happened?" she heard the FBI agent asking.

"I don't know," the man beside the dog sobbed. "He's bleeding!"

"Perhaps he was bitten by a coyote?" the SUEC guard suggested. "There are plenty of those around here, and they can be very aggressive."

"I don't know. A German Shepherd is much larger than a coyote, and could fight them off," the FBI agent said.

"Can I call an ambulance for a dog?" the SUEC guard asked.

"Yes, both San Francisco and San Mateo County have emergency lines. In addition, you can call the Bay Area PET transport, a PET cab that's available 24/7."

Lili was impressed. The FBI was good for something after all.

The agent leaned down to the man beside the dog. "But, if you can carry him, I'd suggest you just take your dog to the animal emergency clinic in Redwood City. You can find the address online. That would be the fastest way to get him there."

"Of course, I can carry him," the man sobbed. "We'll get to the clinic as quickly as possible. He might die!"

"Can you assist?" the FBI agent asked the SUEC guard.

The guard nodded. "Of course. I'll get a vehicle and call the animal hospital to let them know that we're coming."

The SUEC guard ran back to the entrance area. The big man picked up the dog and followed slowly.

The FBI agent stayed back and looked around. He did not see the unconscious man behind the dumpster.

- 40 -

ANNYA

The Assault
Wednesday, May 25, 2033, 10:30 p.m.

A shadow parted from the darkness behind the research building and came towards Annya, Terrel and Dean Hill. It was Heinz with an injured dog in his arms and the SUEC guard at his side. He was weeping uncontrollably.

"What happened?" Annya asked, pity on her face.

"Somebody assaulted my dog," Heinz cried. "He needs a hospital. I'm afraid he might die!"

Annya stepped closer. The dog was eerily calm. She examined him. It helped that they knew each other by now. The dog looked at her with suspicion but did allow her to touch him.

"He has a few broken ribs," she concluded. "He is in pain now, but unless he has major internal injuries, I believe he will recover."

"I know he's in pain!" Heinz exclaimed. "Look at him. He does not even have the strength to howl any more. He does not deserve this. He's the most peaceful, gentle, loving soul in the world. What kind of psychopath hits a dog like that? Somebody tried to poison him, drown him, and beat him to death. This is too much!"

Schnitzel closed his eyes, leaning his big square head against his dad's chest. A bone on his right chest stood up at an unusual angle. He did not move.

Annya felt sorry for both of them. But there was not much she could do. She did not have dog pain medicine in her pocket.

The SUEC guard ran down the street and re-emerged with an electric vehicle. "Please come here, Mr. Tremblay," he called. "I'll bring you to the animal hospital."

Heinz got into the car, and the three left.

Where was Angus? Annya was just about to walk behind the building to look for him when he appeared with an injured SUEC guard in his arms. The guard had a large wound on the back of his head that was bleeding heavily, and he was unconscious.

"Oh, my god!" the Dean exclaimed. "What happened to him?"

Annya looked around. "Where's the person who did this?" she asked.

"We lost him or her in the darkness," Angus said. "Two other guards started the search, and I requested more back up."

"Looks like we could need it," Annya said in a grim voice. "Can you put him down on the bench here?"

Angus complied, and Annya started immediately to provide emergency care. Fortunately, the skull was not deformed; there were no sunken areas, and no visible bone fragments. It was a superficial injury and did not penetrate the skull to reach the brain. Annya did not attempt to clean out the wound. That would be done later in the hospital.

She instructed Angus to call an ambulance. She explained that the scalp contained abundant blood vessels, and that the injury could lead to serious blood loss. She had a stack of sterile gauze in her pocket. She unpacked it, placed it on the wound, and applied steady pressure. The gauze initially soaked through with dark red blood, but then, the bleeding slowly subsided.

The guard opened his eyes. He was somewhat disoriented at first but did not seem to have major neurological issues. He had been lucky. Annya reminded him to stay calm and not move.

This was particularly challenging when they heard gunshots coming from the building.

Terrel asked the Dean to step aside, then pulled his gun and stepped into the building. Angus and three SUEC guards followed him.

The injured guard on the bench wanted to rise, but Annya held him back, keeping her hand on the wound. She assured the man that the FBI would take care of the situation. They would get whatever situation they found under control. Hopefully.

In the distance, she heard the wailing sound of an ambulance siren. It came closer and closer. A white van with flashing lights stopped with squeaking wheels in front of the research building. Two paramedics jumped out. A small crowed had reassembled on the sidewalk and watched them as Annya waved with her free hand. The paramedics rushed to them, examined the injured man, placed him on a stretcher, and moved him into the van.

Annya sighed as the ambulance took off. At least one victim had been saved. The operation was moving in the right direction.

- 41 -

LILI

The Revenge
Wednesday, May 25, 2033, 10:30 p.m.

Lili stepped back from her office window. A woman out there had assaulted a dog and a SUEC guard, stolen the gun from the guard, and was now walking around the building somewhere.

Lili had to notify the security team, but she did not trust Agent Weber. She would inform Terrel Wright.

She stepped into the adjacent imaging lab and searched for her iPhone. Where was that again? In her pocket. She looked for Terrel's number.

There was a buzzing sound at the main entrance of the research building. Someone was entering the building. Lili held out the phone and tiptoed to the door that led to the hall. It was composed of non-magnetic metal to shield people from the MRI scanners in the imaging lab. There was a small window at eye level that allowed her to peek into the foyer. She heard thudding, forceful steps on the marble floor. *Click-tap-tap. Click-tap-tap.*

The small window in the door limited her view. The space in front of her was empty. Sparkling rays of moonlight descended from the cupola like dazzling dancers in a fairytale. There were footsteps coming from the entrance, somewhat asymmetrically. Women's shoes. A young woman in ripped jeans emerged in the hall in front of her. She wore the guard's SUEC cap and jacket.

Lili gasped. The woman's posture, long silky hair and ripped jeans gave her away. It was Ingrid. No doubt it was her. Her right hand and right foot were bandaged. She was limping and using a golf club as a crutch, and a trail of dark marks formed behind her on the freshly cleaned limestone floor.

What were these spots? Lili pressed her face against the small window in her door to see better. Blood! Ingrid was bleeding! What had happened to her, and what did she want here?

Ingrid stopped and looked around. Lili quickly cowered behind the door. Had Ingrid seen her?

After a while, the footsteps continued. *Click-tap-tap. Click-tap-tap.* Lili waited until the sound faded, then looked through the window again. Ingrid was walking up the stairwell. Where was she heading?

Lili pulled her cell phone again and texted Agent Terrel Wright. *Shooter in the building. Ingrid. Second Floor.*

Then, she slowly opened the door of the imaging lab and stepped into the foyer. She heard the footsteps in the hallway above her. She rushed towards the stairs and up to the second floor. At the entrance to the second-floor hallway, she slowed down and listened. The hallway was minimally lit by the dim blue glow of LED lights that lined the skirting board. Bright neon light was coming from Dr. Robinson's office at the end of the hallway. Was he there? *What does Ingrid want?*

Lili felt her heart pounding. She tiptoed closer. Her oversized shadow accompanied her on the wall to her right. The *caw* of a raven outside gave her the chills. Lili cowered behind the post of the infinity sculpture beside the lab entrance. She heard Dr. Robinson's voice. "Hello, Ingrid, you are back?"

Ingrid responded, "Yes."

"Have you been treated at the hospital? I thought that you needed intravenous antibiotics."

"I have been treated and discharged. I am…"

The humming sound of the cryostat compressors in the lab swallowed some of the conversation. Lili leaned closer to the lab entrance and peeked around the corner.

Ingrid stood a few meters away, her back to Lili. Dr. Robinson stood in his office door, relaxed and smiling at her, as usual. "Is that so?" he said. "I received a call that you got involved in a fight in an apartment building on campus. What happened?"

"I found a copy of the list. It was saved on a memory stick. I destroyed it."

Lili noted Dr. Robinson's eyes wandering to the entrance. She leaped back. Had he spotted her? Or her shadow?"

"Hm," he said. "And you came here to tell me that? You could have called."

"The FBI is investigating the case. Your phone is likely tapped," she said. "I wanted to talk with you in person about a different issue."

"And what is that?"

"You did not include me as an author on the patent for preimplantation genetic testing," Ingrid said with a shaking voice.

Dr. Robinson looked at her with his piercing blue eyes. "No, I did not," he responded calmly.

"*I* did all the work for it!"

"Ingrid, a patent is about intellectual property. It was my idea. That's what the patent is about. You just executed the work."

"*I just* executed the work?" she responded in a high-pitched voice. "I did *all* of the work! You needed scientific data to support the patent claim. There would be no patent without my work. In fact, I worked around the clock for this! It is mine!"

"You do not need to worry about your future, Ingrid. You will become the leader of this lab."

"So that I can do *more* work for you? And you'll walk away with your pockets full of cash? I don't think that works for me," she said in a shaky, rage-filled voice.

"Ingrid, you're overreacting. Remember, I am your father. I want the best for you."

Ingrid spat in his direction. "You want the best for yourself. You gave your sperm away for money. And then you exploited me for money!"

"Ingrid, calm down. I will always watch out for you!"

"Watching out like not adding me to a patent that monetizes my work?" she said in a scathing voice. "Well, I can take better care of myself."

Ingrid reached into her pocket and pointed the gun at Dr. Robinson. Lili held her breath.

Dr. Robinson raised his arms. "Ingrid, don't do anything stupid. We can work this out. What would you like me to do instead?"

Ingrid looked at him with a pinched face. "Did you sell the patent?"

"I did."

"Excellent. Then, I will inherit the income from my daddy, who unfortunately committed suicide."

Lili looked around. Where was Terrel?

She noted the golf club leaning against the inner door frame. She got up and walked through the door, her index finger over her mouth. Dr. Robinson looked at her briefly. He did not say a word. Ingrid's back was to her.

Lili grabbed the club, stepped towards the closest lab bench, and crawled underneath. Her heart raced. Ingrid had a gun. But she was too agitated to notice her.

Lili slowly crept closer under the cover of the bench. Perhaps she could leap forward and knock her unconscious. She tightened her grip.

- 42 -

LILI

How I Feel
Wednesday, May 25, 2033, 11:00 p.m.

Lili tried to crawl closer to Ingrid under the cover of the lab desk. Ingrid was aiming the gun at Dr. Robinson.

Suddenly, a black man stepped into the room. It was Mr. Johnes, Nia's father. "YOU killed my daughter," he cried with a shaking voice.

Dr. Robinson looked at the man. "I did not kill your daughter," he said calmly.

Ingrid looked over her shoulder at the old man, then back at Dr. Robinson, still pointing the gun at him. "Nia did this to herself," Ingrid said with a trembling voice. "She wanted to sabotage our work. Oliver and I were creating a new generation of humans—people who would not suffer from infections. People who would be stronger than bacteria and viruses. Nia was unable to see this."

"Did you kill your sister?" the man cried.

"Nia was not my sister. She was an experiment gone wrong— the DNA of a genius merged with a stupid mother. Out came a stupid girl."

"You will not call my wife and daughter stupid!" Mr. Johnes exclaimed between clenched teeth. He extended his right arm, and Lili gasped. He had a gun as well.

Ingrid looked back at the old man. "I'm sorry. I'm just trying to explain," she said. "Nia had no appreciation for the great science that led to her existence."

"And so, you killed her?"

Ingrid shrugged. "I told you: I asked her to stay away from our project, but she did not listen. Her life was sacrificed for the advancement of humanity."

"*You* did this!"

Nia's father pointed the gun at Ingrid.

Dr. Robinson raised his hands. "Wait!" He looked at Lili.

Lili held her breath and cowered deeper under her desk. Would he reveal her to the shooter? Sweat ran down her back.

Dr. Robinson's gaze went to the golf club in her hand. He was trying to communicate that she should use it, but she was scared. How should she bring down two shooters at once? Impossible.

Dr. Robinson looked back at the man with the gun.

"It wasn't Ingrid," he said to Mr. Johnes. "It was Mr. Jacub Bezdomny, the building manager. He committed suicide earlier this evening."

Mr. Johnes's face only grew grimmer. "*You* keep your mouth shut," he replied in a cold voice. "I saw Nia's notes about your gene games. *You*, of all people, should have protected her." He leveled the gun at Dr. Robinson.

"*I* am already shooting him," Ingrid shouted with a trembling voice. Lili wasn't sure if Ingrid was angry or anxious.

"Okay, go ahead," the man said calmly.

Ingrid looked at Dr. Robinson, the gun trembling in her hands. "Don't do anything stupid," he whispered. "I am your father. I love you!"

There were footsteps on the stairs and voices in the hallway. "This way!"

Lili held her breath. It was Terrel's voice. He was coming.

"You are no father. You are a predator!" Mr. Johnes exclaimed.

Lili could hardly grasp what happened in the next split-second. Mr. Johnes aimed at Dr. Robinson. There was a thudding sound. Ingrid spun around and jumped towards Nia's father. Sprays of blood flew through the air. The smell of gun powder filled the room.

Ingrid stumbled, raising her arms. Then she fell forward to the ground.

"Ingrid!" Dr. Robinson cried out. He jumped forward, kneeled in front of her, grabbed her shoulders, and pulled her to his chest. She made some gargling noises.

Nia's father looked at the professor and raised the gun again. "You made her kill my daughter!"

Lili was shocked. She had never seen anyone kill someone right in front of her. Blood soaked through Ingrid's silver jacket, penetrating the large white SUEC signs on her chest like diabolic fingers. Ingrid fell back into Dr. Robinson's arms, near-lifeless.

Lili tightened her grip around the golf club. She was horrified. But she also had to stop this madness.

The footsteps in the hallway became louder. Dr. Robinson looked at the door as a sharp voice filled the room. "Don't move."

A black man in an FBI jacket entered, both arms extended, pointing a gun at Nia's father. It was FBI Agent Terrel Wright. Behind him, Agent Weber and two SUEC guards followed, all pointing guns at Mr. Johnes.

Nia's father looked briefly back at them. Then he turned back to Dr. Robinson, refocusing his gun on him. "Shoot if you want," he said. "I have nothing to lose. But this guy will die first."

"Mr. Johnes, don't make any mistake," Terrel said calmly. "I can see that Ingrid has a gun in her hand. You were defending yourself. But shooting an unarmed man is a felony. *We* will bring him to justice."

"No, you won't," Mr. Johnes responded. "I have seen your justice system. Rich white men like him always walk away. Not today."

Lili looked at Terrel. She could help. She cowered under the bench just an arm's length behind Nia's father. She took all her courage and swung the golf club as forcefully as she could into Mr. Johnes's ankles. He cried out in pain and stumbled forward as three bullets passed over his head and hit the window frame in front of him.

A second later, Terrel leaped against him. Both men crashed onto the floor, their guns thrown across the room. They grappled briefly, but the young FBI agent was much stronger than the old man. Terrel grabbed Mr. Johnes's arms and cuffed him.

At the same time, Agent Weber jumped towards Lili, pulled her out from underneath the bench, and cuffed her as well. "I helped you!" she protested.

Terrel nodded. "She saved Mr. Johnes's life," he said.

"We will see about that," Agent Weber said grimly. "This golf club was used to assault an SUEC agent outside."

"Ingrid brought the golf club here," Lili protested.

"And Lili texted us to come here," Terrel added.

"We will get this all straightened out once everyone here has been interviewed," Agent Weber said. He pointed at Oliver Stuart Robinson. "…including Dr. Robinson."

Oliver still kneeled on the ground, tears streaming down his face. He had carefully lifted Ingrid's body and was rocking her in his arms. She looked back at him without saying a word. A gush of bright red blood formed on the left side of chest. She coughed, and her gaze started to fade. Oliver clutched her to his chest. "Stay with me, Ingrid," he begged. "Don't go!"

She looked at him. "I wish I had a father who cared for me," she whispered.

"I do care for you!" Oliver cried out. "I do! You are exactly the daughter I've always dreamed of, Ingrid! I love you!"

Ingrid looked at him with a faint smile. Her face got paler and paler. "Maybe," she slurred. Then, her head fell back.

"No!" Dr. Robinson exclaimed. He looked at his daughter, tears streaming down his face.

Then he jumped up and grabbed Mr. Johnes by his collar. "What did you do?" he cried as Agent Weber stepped forward and pulled him back.

"Now you know how I feel," the old man said coldly.

- 43 -

ANNYA

The Arrest
Wednesday, May 25, 2033, 11:30 p.m.

The door of the research building opened, and Terrel stepped out, guiding an elderly man in handcuffs. After him came Angus Weber with Lili, also in handcuffs, and two SUEC guards, who flanked Oliver Robinson on each side.

Annya shook her head at seeing the Black man and the Asian woman in handcuffs, and the white man escorted without any restraint.

She rushed to Angus. "Did you get the shooter?" she asked.

He pointed at Terrel. "Terrel got him. I'm afraid Mr. Johnes played vigilante."

"Why is Lili in handcuffs?" she asked. "She found the shooter and called you."

"She was holding the golf club that injured the SUEC guard. He was an undercover federal agent," Angus responded calmly.

Annya shook her head. "Lili would not harm anyone. I'm sure there's a good explanation."

"Ingrid came in with the golf club," Lili explained. "She leaned it against the wall when she reached for her gun. I thought I had to stop her, so I picked it up."

"What did Ingrid want in the building?" Annya asked.

"She wanted to shoot Dr. Robinson." Lili pointed at the professor, who had been unusually quiet.

"I'm afraid Ingrid was mentally ill," he said in a hoarse voice. "I didn't realize that until today. She was obsessed with her research. She engaged in illegal activities by infecting people with bacteria or viruses and testing their ability to recover. Nia threatened to report her to the university authorities, which would have gotten Ingrid fired, so she killed her."

"Didn't you state earlier today that the building manager was the suspect?" Terrel asked.

Dr. Robinson cleared his throat. "Jacub Bezdomny found out that Ingrid infected people who were conceived in our IVF clinic and who all carried a mutation of the CCR5 gene. So, she killed him too."

Lili's jaw dropped. "So, you were a victim?" she exclaimed in disbelief.

Dr. Robinson nodded. "Nia gave a thumb drive with a list of the infected people to Heinz Tremblay. Ingrid destroyed the memory stick and tried to kill Heinz. Then she came for me because I had started to uncover her activities."

"She was upset because you did not include her in your patent!" Lili cried out.

"Careful, folks," Angus Weber intervened. "The evidence will be collected and provided to the court."

"*He* was the mastermind behind everything!" Mr. Johnes shouted with a pinched face, his mouth twisted into a snarl. "*He* used that woman to do his dirty work. *He* told her to kill my daughter."

Dr. Robinson looked at him. "Mr. Johnes, I am very sorry for your loss" he said calmly. "But be careful not to make any false allegations here. I could sue you for defamation."

Mr. Johnes spat at Dr. Robinson. "I hope you rot in hell!"

"We will untangle this, Mr. Johnes," Terrel interjected. "Remember that anything you say can be used against you in court. You have the right to talk to a lawyer for advice before you say anything or before we ask you any questions. If you cannot afford a lawyer, one will be appointed for you if you wish."

Mr. Johnes clenched his teeth.

A black Ford van with FBI signs arrived in front of the research building. The driver got out and opened the sliding door to the back cabin. Terrel and Mr. Johnes got in, and the two FBI agents followed with Dr. Robinson.

Terrel turned to Angus. "Dr. Lili Pham helped us tremendously. I don't think she's a threat to anyone. I certainly agree that she should be interrogated as well, but I think we can uncuff her." He pointed at the spectators at the other side of the street. "It would send the right message. Remember, Dr. Pham has to return to work here."

Agent Weber nodded and turned to Annya. "Annya, will you serve as Dr. Pham's guard? You'll have to come with us anyways to provide your witness statement. If you agree, I will release her handcuffs."

Annya nodded. "Of course."

Agent Weber uncuffed Lili's hands. "I understand that you helped significantly with the resolution of this case. How do I say thank you in your language?"

Lili looked at him in surprise. "That would be, *'Thank you.'*"

- 44 -

HEINZ

The Celebration
Saturday, May 28, 2033, 2:00 p.m.

Heinz Tremblay and Schnitzel arrived at the tall Spanish-flavored home in Atherton where Dean Robert Hill and his husband, Atharv Patel, lived. It was a part of the town that actually had sidewalks and middle-sized houses without big gates, as other areas of the town were famous for. Heinz marveled at the beautiful stucco façade and rounded gable of Dean Hill's house.

He parked his 2003 Jeep Liberty under an olive tree on the spacious front porch and helped Schnitzel out. The dog whined softly as Heinz lifted him off the back seat and placed him carefully on the ground. Schnitzel limped with his dad to the arched double leaf entrance, carefully avoiding any pressure on his casted right hind leg. The veterinary team had diagnosed several broken ribs and a broken femur as a result of the assault with the golf club. The femur fracture had been fixed with an orthopedic plate, but the ribs had to heal by themselves. Fortunately, Schnitzel had not encountered an injury to the head, like the SUEC guard. The poor man had suffered a severe concussion and was still in the hospital.

Heinz rang the doorbell. Footsteps approached from inside the building, and Atharv opened the door. "Great to see you, Heinz," he said with a broad smile. "I'm so glad you could make it." He stepped aside with an inviting gesture.

Heinz and Schnitzel stepped into a marble floor entryway with a high ceiling and exposed wooden beams. It smelled of freshly grilled meat. Schnitzel held his nuzzle high and followed the scent with a wagging tail. Heinz and Atharv laughed as they walked to a slanted ornate oak door at the end of the entryway. They started to hear chattering voices and piano music. "How is your dog?" Atharv asked.

"He is slowly recovering. It will take some time for the fractures to heal, but he's doing better every day, and his vet expects a full recovery."

"I am so glad to hear that!"

They entered a light-infused sunroom at the back of the house. The tall wall-to-wall windows provided a view of a large, tropical garden with palm trees, ferns, and white orchids. People in expensive-looking suits and cocktail dresses were standing in small groups or sitting on white-cushioned teak seats, engaged in lively discussions. Dean Hill was standing in a small group in the left corner of the room, holding a baby girl in an adorable teddy bear jumpsuit.

Heinz walked over to him. "Congratulations on your baby," he said. The baby looked at him with alert, deep blue eyes. Schnitzel lifted his nose to explore the unusual scent of a newborn human.

"Thank you!" Dean Hill responded with a broad smile.

Atharv joined them, placing his arm around Robert's shoulders. "Isn't she adorable?" he said. "We are so in love!"

"What is her name?" Heinz asked.

"We called her Hope. We thought it was appropriate. She is our hope for a better future—a future where people will be more tolerant, more accepting of each other, and less violent," Dean Hill said.

"That is a beautiful name, and she already lives up to it!" Heinz looked at the cute little girl, who smiled at him. Schnitzel nuzzled his leg to remind him of his existence, and Heinz ruffled his head.

"Congrats to your new family member!" Terrel Wright joined the group.

"Thank you, Agent Wright," Dean Hill responded. "I am so glad we can focus on the pleasant aspects of life again."

"Was the shooter convicted?" Heinz asked.

"Our investigations have confirmed that Mrs. Maulvi murdered Nia Johnes. Several witnesses independently reported her confession. We do not have enough information about Mr. Bezdomny's death, but we assume that Mrs. Maulvi was responsible for his death as well. Mr. Johnes is currently in custody and will face a trial in a few weeks. Since Mrs. Maulvi had a gun in the encounter with him, his attorney will plead for self-defense."

"What about Dr. Robinson?" Heinz asked.

"He might have been involved, but we could not find any evidence to prove it, so he has been released."

"But he manipulated human embryos?" Heinz asked.

"It seems that he *selected* embryos with a certain genetic trait. Unfortunately, preimplantation genetic diagnosis is not regulated in the United States. Dr. Robinson stated that he only performed routine genetic screening tests to exclude hereditary diseases. According to him, an enrichment of the CCR5delta32 gene in his patients is a pure coincidence."

"I see." Heinz pointed at Lili, who was chatting with her husband Mark and Aiko Tanaka, the Dean's administrative assistant, at the other end of the room. "And Dr. Lili Pham has been released as well?"

"Yes," Terrel confirmed. "There was no wrongdoing on her part. In fact, she helped us tremendously, and she probably saved Mr. Johnes's life through her brave actions." He turned to Dean Hill. "Dr. Pham is exceptionally smart, full of integrity, and empathetic—great qualities for a leader, if you ask me."

"Duly noted," Dean Hill responded. "I have her on a shortlist for a Vice Dean post. Her and Dr. Annya Segond, if she is available." He pointed at Annya, who was talking with Agent Angus Weber outside on a small porch in front of the sunroom that led to the garden.

"Are the two an item?" Atharv asked with a mischievous smile.

"Not officially," Terrel responded. "But what is not can still be."

Their conversation was interrupted by multiple *buzz* tones of incoming text messages. Multiple guests reached for their phones.

Dean Hill looked at his phone and then at his husband with wide-open eyes. "Honey, I believe I need to tell you something," he said in a stammering voice. "Could we talk privately for a moment?"

Heinz's phone blinked as well—it was an anonymous message with an attached photo. He opened it and started to laugh. This was hilarious!

Terrel looked at Heinz, then at the Dean. "You didn't step down?"

The Dean shook his head. "No, I did not. I was hoping that the threat would dissipate. Dr. Robinson submitted his resignation under the condition that he could keep his patent. I agreed, so I thought the issue was solved."

Dean Hill looked at his husband. "Honey, could we have a word in private, please?"

Atharv patted Robert Hill's shoulder. "Robby, I am the chief information technology officer here. Do you really believe that anyone could embarrass my husband with an e-message?"

Robert looked at him with wide-open eyes. "I don't understand."

People around him stared at their phones and started to laugh as well.

"Look what we got here," Atharv pulled his iPhone and opened the message. It showed a photo of two men with bare chests in a hotel bed. One was a beautiful white man with curly blonde hair and Greek features. The other was Dr. Robinson.

"What the deuce?" Robert Hill exclaimed.

Heinz laughed. "Let me guess. Photoshop?"

"Exactly!" Atharv responded with a proud smile.

"I did not hear any of this conversation," Terrel chuckled. He offered Heinz his arm, and they both walked to Lili's group with Schnitzel in tow. Lili greeted them with a toast.

- 45 -

CHRISTINA

Arc of Justice
Saturday, May 28, 2033, 7:00 p.m.

Cristina had made herself comfortable on her couch. All of her colleagues and friends were at the Dean's party, but she did not feel like celebrating. She still mourned Nia's and Jacub's death, and she was deeply disturbed that Oliver Robinson got away. *He* had been the mastermind behind all evil. *He* had played with unborn babies genes to create upgraded humans, people who would be resistant to infections. He had not asked the parents for permission, nor did he care about unintended consequences. Perhaps these gene-manipulated people had a higher risk of getting cancer, or they lived less long than ordinary humans. Only time would tell. Nia had been so smart. She had uncovered the entire gene manipulation business, when everyone else had no clue what was really going on in Oliver's lab. And then Oliver had incited Ingrid to kill her half-sister. And her half-brother. Oh, Oliver could be so persuasive when he wanted something. Cristina knew this from her own experience. Ingrid had been his puppet. She had infected Olivers human creations with bacteria, viruses and fungi, to test the results of their human experiment. She had killed Nia and framed Jacub for murder when he started to uncover the truth. Ingrid would have done anything for Oliver. And she had been jealous of Cristina. The only woman for whom Oliver had publicly shown some feelings. Ingrid had been jealous and tried to frame Cristina for kidnapping her and drowning an innocent dog in her apartment. She wanted to get Cristina out of the way and take her place. Ingrid had longed for Oliver's love and acceptance. She could not know that a narcist was not able to give what she needed most. A father-less girl trying to nurture her soul in a cruel world. Cristina felt pity for Ingrid – and guilt about her death. She remembered her conversation with

Terrel Wright. He had invited her to try to curse someone and see if it materialized in the real world. She remembered exactly what she had said: "*I wish that the person who ordered Nia's murder would feel the same pain as her parents are feeling right now.*"

And then Oliver's daughter had been killed. Was it her fault? Cristina had been raised to believe that religion was good—higher morale, integrity, salvation—but it only led to destruction. Some people left the church because they did not believe any more. And others left because they were just disappointed. Ingrid was dead and Oliver was walking around. That's not what Cristina had meant with her cry for justice. Neither God nor the FBI had taken Oliver to his deserved sentence. The hand had died, and the mastermind lived unharmed. She had been wrong. Cristina would never curse anyone again. The spiritual world was the realm of the gods. Humans should focus on the physical world. She sipped on her wine. If fate wanted her to intervene, then she needed a sign.

The doorbell rang.
Who was that? She was not expecting anyone.
The doorbell rang again.
Cristina got up. She walked to the entrance and opened the door.
It was him, in his leather jacket and worn-out jeans, looking at her with his steel-blue eyes. He looked a little tired, his hair messed-up by the afternoon wind. "I heard that husband of yours got lost," he said with a faint smile. "And I saw an opportunity here to offer my company."

He stood there awkwardly, hands in his pockets, looking at her. His blue eyes were all she could see.

"Oliver, we have been there before," she said calmly. "I cannot approve of your business. It is against everything I believe. Go home."

"I have some news that you might like to hear. Can I come in?"

Cristina shook her head. "I am grieving my lost friends – and if you stay another minute, there is a good chance that I will kill you."

He looked at her with his intense gaze. "I quit."

She stared at him. "You did what?"

"I quit. I cannot continue this work after Ingrid's death. I have enough money to live off from the interest of my patents. I want to work a lot less and have more fun. Will you join me?"

He spread his arms.

This man was just too much. All she wanted and despised in one person. She hesitated for a moment. Then, she went in. They kissed passionately. Another resident came down the aisle and looked at them in surprise. They laughed at each other, amused, as if they were both in on a joke that the rest of the world did not understand.

Cristina pulled Oliver into the room and closed the door. She ran her fingers through his hair, down his body. He lifted her up and carried her to the bedroom.

***

The sun plunged with dark orange and red colors behind the redwood forest. He was standing on the balcony, enjoying a cigarette while Cristina fixed a quick dinner in the kitchen. He smiled. Life was good.

He pulled his phone and saw the annoying photo. His plan to embarrass Dean Hill had failed, but it did not matter. He had other plans now. And what a ridiculous idea it had been to photoshop him into the picture. Nobody would believe that he had interest in male company. Even Cristina had found it funny—a student prank. It would blow over like a breeze.

His phone blinked with a text message from Nathanael Zhang, CEO of OrchidBio. Oliver looked through the glass window of the balcony door. The door was only half-closed, but Cristina was busy. He dialed Nathanael's number. "Hi, Nathanael, what's up?"

"Oliver, I just got the confirmation that your lab can be transferred to the University of Shanghai. The team there will be very excited to work with you."

"That sounds great! I'm glad it worked out!"

"I heard you quit your job at SUEC. We do need your expertise. An alliance between OrchidBio and your team is crucial for our success."

"Don't worry. My son Larry will take over the lab. He will collaborate with you. I'll stay in the background."

"That sounds great! I remember your son was not that interested in working in the lab. How did you convince him otherwise?"

"I did not have to do anything. He worked a few gruesome 24/7 shifts as an attending physician. After that, a career as a physician–scientist sounded much more attractive to him. And the salary bonus, of course. He is a great kid. I'm sure you will enjoy working with him."

"I look forward to it. But we also need *your* input as well. You are one of a kind, you know that?"

"No worries! I will come to visit you in Shanghai. How about next month? Or is that too early?"

"It's perfect! Your new lab there will be ready by then. I'll ask my assistant to arrange flights, and we can all meet there."

"Excellent! See you there!"

Oliver smiled. The world was a wonderful place. All the stars had aligned in his favor after all.

He walked back into the kitchen. Cristina smiled at him and handed him a glass of champagne. He cheered and took a sip. Then, he pulled her close and kissed her. She turned around, reached for two plates, forks, and knives, and pointed at the living room. "We need to eat. Can you place these on the table?"

"Of course, lady boss!" He kissed her again, grabbed the champagne glass and the plates, and walked over to the dining table. He took another sip. And another. The sparkles felt good on his tongue and went straight up to his head. All the stress from the last few days evaporated. Time to celebrate. Oliver took another sip. He felt a little dizzy. Had Cristina added some vodka or something? Oliver steadied himself at the table. His knees became weak. Then, he slipped to the ground.

***

Cristina waited a few more minutes. It was eerie calm in her apartment. Her heart beats were pounding up to her ears. She had never done anything like this. But it was her duty. A few drops of cyanide in his champagne. For Nia. And Jacub. And Ingrid. They deserved justice for being exploited and slayed by this man. Cristina waited a few more minutes. Then, she bent down and palpated Oliver's pulse. Nothing. She sighed. She had liked how he had made her feel. Special, smart, beautiful. But his demise would benefit all of humanity. No more gene games. At least for now. Cristina was not so naïve to think that she could prevent human engineering from taking over the future. But perhaps she could slow it down a bit.

She pulled her cell phone and called 911. Then she texted Annya: *Oliver came to see me. He broke down in my apartment. No pulse. Perhaps a heart attack. I called 911.*

A message from Annya came back instantly. *I am at the Dean's party with Angus. We will be there in about 15 minutes.*

Cristina put the phone away and sat down. The arc of the universe was long. But it always bent towards justice. If a courageous human pulled it in the right direction.

ACKNOWLEDGMENTS

I am grateful for many people who helped me writing this novel. Many thanks to my students and colleagues who shared their insights with me about positive and negative interactions in the academic environment. You helped me creating authentic multi-facetted scenes of the academic world inspired by real-life experiences. To everyone who contributed to this book directly or indirectly, thank you!

I would like to specifically thank my awesome husband, Dr. Thomas Link. From planning the plot to reading early drafts and giving me advice on how to build suspense, Thomas provided important input for this story. Many thanks to my colleagues Dr. Ann Leong, Dr. Kristen Yeom, and Dr. Marta Flory for contributing expertise and insights on infectious diseases, along with pictures of medical imaging studies for the medical-educational version of this book.

I am grateful to my colleagues from the Pegasus Medical Writing Group at Stanford for reading the first chapters and offering their critical feedback on the overall roadmap and character development. I am also grateful to Lauren Schoenthaler for providing important input regarding the legal aspects of writing a detective story that is set in a medical environment. Many thanks to Elisabeth Daldrup and Berthold Schroeter for taking the time to read the final book draft and providing me with valuable feedback on the reader experience.

A very special thanks goes out to my editor Oren Eades for his excellent, accurate and efficient work. Oren pays attention to every detail, and he never stops striving to be the best. I'm very grateful to him for his thorough analysis of the manuscript, his helpful editorial remarks, and his constructive comments, which improved the quality of the final product.

A big thanks to Paul Palmer-Edwards for designing the cover art for this book. Paul took the time to read the entire book before designing several insightful visual representations of its content. I used one here and will use another for the upcoming German translation of this book. I am also very grateful for expert advice by David Carriere on publicizing the book in magazines, newspapers, radio and social media outlets. Many thanks also to Hendrik Daldrup for helping with the creation of the book's website, which effectively connects our publishing team with interested readers.

And last but not least, I would like to thank you, the reader, for reading this book and engaging in reflections on identity and ethical questions in medical research. I hope that the experiences conveyed in this book will make you stronger when you encounter micro- or macroaggressions in the academic world such that you can stand up for yourself and others.

ABOUT THE AUTHOR

Elisabeth Link, MD is a Professor of Radiology at Stanford University who lives with her husband Thomas Link, MD, in San Francisco, California. In addition to her work as a physician-scientist, she is member of the Pegasus Physician Writers at Stanford, a group of physicians who write creatively.

Dr. Link first began writing creatively as a child in order to entertain her grandmother, who was living alone in a small house in a forest in Northern Germany. Later, as a young college student, she was surprised that her reflections on human experiences (and that of her beloved dog Bobby) provided her with much welcomed extra income through publications in local newsletters. After completing her medical education, Dr. Link's thirst for exploration led her to emigrate to the United States. While she embraced the career opportunities in the new world, she was curious to understand human interactions and power dynamics at high end academic institutions. The Pegasus Physician Writers group at Stanford provided her with much welcomed support to share her thoughts and experiences on identity and social justice through page turning detective stories.

Throughout her career, Dr. Link passionately contributed to the diversification of the biomedical sciences through tireless advocacy, mentorship and support of women and underrepresented minorities in the field of Science, Technology, Engineering and Mathematics/ Medicine (STEM). Dr. Link is widely known for her powerful reflections and opinion pieces on women in STEM (e.g., "The Fermi Paradox in STEM - Where Are the Women Leaders?" https://doi.org/10.1007/s11307-017-1124-4). Her novels describe strong female protagonists who conquer major obstacles in the academic world and inspire others – male and female - to stand up for themselves and face their own challenges. Dr. Link received more than 50 honors and awards for her creative works over the past three decades, but the feedback from her students is most rewarding to her, like the note below from one of her mentees:

"I am aware that I cannot control the barriers that enter my life but, like water, I will never be broken. Medicine is an intellectual journey, and I am determined to reach my goal of becoming the best doctor my patients will ever encounter."

A NOTE FOR THE READER

Thank you for reading an authorized copy of this book. Monasteria Press LLC is a company that is subsidized by its entrepreneurial founders. By purchasing our publications, you are supporting our authors and allowing Monasteria Press to continue to publish new books for future readers.

If you would like to read additional books from Monasteria Press, you can find our newest publications on our website: monasteria-press.com
To stay updated about future projects and connect with Dr. Link via email, you can contact editors@monasteria-press.com

In case you liked the story about Nia Johnes, please consider submitting a review about the book on Amazon, Barnes & Noble, Powell's, Goodreads, or Twitter. Reviews are very important. They help to spread the word about great books and can make an author's day. A great review is a wonderful reward for the hard work, long weekends, and sleepless nights that the author has invested to share their story. While we appreciate your enthusiastic support, please remember not to give away the entire plot and to allow other readers the courtesy of having some surprises.

Thank you for being part of our amazing community! We look forward to welcoming you back soon!

The Monasteria Press Team

BOOKS BY ELISABETH LINK

Who Killed Nia Johnes?
A Tale for Healthcare Professionals

Elisabeth Link, MD
Monasteria Press 2022

A mystery novel for medical students, nursing students and other trainees in the medical field. In the secluded Silicon Valley University of Evolutionary Computation (SUEC), a young researcher, Dr. Nia Johnes, is shot by a mysterious killer. The seemingly idyllic university community is turned upside down as FBI special agent Terrel Wright, CIA operative Dr. Annya Segond and radiologist Dr. Lili Pham work together to solve the mystery behind Nia's death. Are the unexplained infections that are plaguing the campus somehow connected? What are the unsettling research activities that the SUEC leaders would prefer to keep quiet? Terrel, Anya and Lili must fight to save their lives and their careers as they race to prevent further deaths and to uncover the shocking truth behind *Who Killed Nia Johnes?*

This special edition of WKNJ includes medical images of infectious diseases that characters in the novel suffer -- showing details that help radiologists rendering a diagnosis. To find Nia's killer, Terrel, Annya and Lili need to analyze x-rays, computed tomography (CT) and magnetic resonance imaging (MRI) scans, uncovering important clues that help them solving the mystery. This is a great read for anyone interested in medical education.

Paperback ISBN 978-1-7372582-9-2
Hardback ISBN 978-1-958277-90-4
eBook ISBN 978-1-958277-99-7

BOOKS BY ELISABETH LINK

The Stolen Brain Chip

Elisabeth Link, MD

Monasteria Press 2021

A fast-paced mystery novel with an educational twist. The story revolves around a fictional university in the hills above Redwood City, CA, known as Silicon Valley University of Evolutionary Computation (SUEC). Newly developed brain chips, which can enhance a person's brain capacity, are stolen. Thus begins a string of events that leaves fifteen people injured, five hospitalized and four dead. Dr. Lili Pham, Dr. Annya Segond, FBI agent Terrel Wright and FBI agent Angus Weber start a race against time to rescue a young student from a ruthless killer, retrieve the brain chips and prevent a bomb explosion at SUEC.

To find the killer before he strikes again, it will take more than traditional on-the-scene evidence. The clues about the murderer revolve around various types of bone fractures that characters in the novel suffer -- pathological details that new medical students and radiologists often have a hard time remembering. Some of the characters suffer specific fractures, which are diagnosed in detail in the book and provide clues to the mysteries of who the killer is and who stole the brain chips. The book also includes X-ray images showing what those different fractures look like. This is a great read for anyone interested in medicine and medical education.

The novel has a strong female protagonist and conveys the concept that we are all heroes-in-waiting. The time will come when each one of us will get a chance to step up and be the hero.

Paperback ISBN 978-1-7372582-3-0
Hardback ISBN 978-1-7372582-5-4
eBook ISBN 978-1-7372582-4-7

Library of Congress Control Number (LCCN) 2021950975

BOOKS BY ELISABETH LINK

The Claim

Elisabeth Link, MD
Monasteria Press 2023

An elite university. An abduction. An FBI investigation.
On October 8, 2033, a young medical insurance agent, Dr. Frieda Ending, was dragged into a van and disappeared without a trace. FBI special agent Angus Weber and CIA operative Dr. Annya Segond launch an investigation that leads them to the hospital of Silicon Valley University of Evolutionary Computation (SUEC) in Redwood City, California, where all pending medical insurance claims for children with cancer were suddenly approved. Who is behind this? Is Frieda a victim or a villain? The only witness is the parrot Caramba who keeps his beak shut. As Annya and Angus delve deeper into the investigation, they uncover a trail of greed and betrayal that leads them closer to the truth, and a finally, a shocking revelation.
The Claim is an insightful and gripping medical mystery novel, which exposes fundamental problems of profit-based medical insurance systems. The game out there is rigged, and everybody knows it.

Coming soon:
Paperback ISBN 978-1-958277-05-8
Hardback ISBN 978-1-958277-07-2
eBook ISBN 978-1-958277-06-5